NURSING PROCESS

Concepts and Application

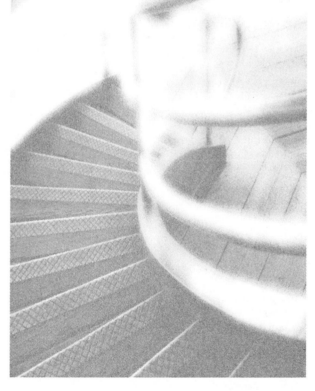

Wanda Wallher Seaback, RN, BSN
Professor of Nursing
Kingwood College
Kingwood, Texas

DELMAR
THOMSON LEARNING™

Australia Canada Mexico Singapore Spain United Kingdom United States

DELMAR

THOMSON LEARNING

Nursing Process: Concepts and Application
by Wanda Wallher Seaback

Business Unit Director: William Brottmiller
Acquisitions Editor: Matthew Filimonov
Development Editor: Darcy M. Scelsi
Executive Marketing Manager: Dawn F. Gerrain
Project Editor: Mary Ellen Cox
Production Coordinator: John Mickelbank
Art/Design Coordinator: Mary Colleen Libardi
Cover: TDB Publishing Service

To my husband, George:
You have encouraged me to reach for the stars.
Thank you for your patience and love.

To my children, Phillip, Candi, Lori, and Nicholas:
Believe in yourself. Be true to those you love.

To my grandchildren, Brooke, Breanne, and Jacob:
You have renewed the child in me and made my heart soar with pride.

To my respected friend and mentor, Vicki Pruitt:
You are an inspiration to the many lives you have touched.

To my colleagues, Thelma Bowie, Carol Erb,
Suzanne Gates, Carol Goldsby,
Linda King, Margarita Knox, Lore Porter,
and Marybeth Sinclair:
Without your support and encouragement,
this project would not have been possible.

My heartfelt thanks to you all.

NOTICE TO THE READER

Table of Contents

Preface

Nursing Process: Concepts and Application was written with the *educator* and *student* in mind. The student's manual is written and arranged to correspond with the educator's presentation material, thus promoting interactive learning and stimulating student questions and in-class discussion.

The nursing process is one of the most important concepts to be taught in fundamental nursing. Most theory presented in nursing textbooks is based on the nursing process steps: assessment, problem identification/diagnosis, planning and outcome identification, implementation, and evaluation. National licensing examination questions are formatted and written utilizing the nursing process steps.

This interactive student textbook coincides with the educator's presentation material, and numerous activities are included to clarify instruction and to provide practice for the student. Activities are necessary for students to understand the presented concepts and theory and for practical application of these concepts. The appendices include a complete current list of NANDA nursing diagnoses for easy reference. The student's workbook is written in a format designed to make learning fun, and, once the workbook is completed, it becomes an important reference for the student to use throughout nursing education.

Key Features:
- The interactive student text and the educator presentations are linked so that the student can follow along completing the text and interacting in the class discussion.
- Text presents the nursing process in an easy-to-understand, step-by-step format.
- Student Practice activities promote application of the concept behind each step.
- Student Practice activities build upon one another, increasing in complexity to promote understanding, critical thinking, and practical application of each step of the nursing process.
- Numerous examples and cases allow students to apply their knowledge as they progress through the text.

THE AUTHOR'S CONCEPT

In developing this textbook, I desired a work that could be adapted to all levels of nursing education, beginning with vocational/practical, applied science/associate degree nursing, and then broadening concepts and theory to embrace baccalaureate nursing. I believed it was important to present essential material students must learn and understand in order to apply the nursing process in clinical practice.

I was motivated to compose an instruction manual with an accompanying student workbook, providing important basic information and laying a foundation, step-by-step, that each student could understand and apply. Since its initial development in 1996, a great deal of the content has been rewritten and revised for clarity and effectiveness to benefit students' understanding. I was pleased to find my nursing students through the use of this text, were finally able to understand the concepts and demonstrated the ability to apply their knowledge to clinical practice. My students consistently demonstrate an overall improvement in critical thinking and clinical application through the use of this text. *Nursing Process: Concepts and Application* is the culmination of this endeavor.

Nursing Process: An Overview

"Everyday sanitary knowledge, or the knowledge of nursing, or in other words, of how to put the constitution in such a state as that it will have no disease, or that it can recover from disease, takes a higher place. It is recognized as the knowledge which every one ought to have—distinct from medical knowledge, which only a profession can have.

The reparative process which Nature has instituted and which we will call disease has been hindered by some want of knowledge or attention, in one or in all of these things, and pain, suffering, or interruption of the whole process sets in.

. . . nothing but observation and experience will teach us the ways to maintain or to bring back the state of health."

Florence Nightingale

OBJECTIVES

Upon completion of this chapter, the student should be able to:

- Describe the historical evolution of the nursing process.
- Discuss the nursing process as a therapeutic framework and describe how it is accepted as a tool for promoting multidisciplinary collaboration.
- List and define the five steps of the nursing process.
- Identify theories and philosophies nursing professionals use in practice to gain an understanding of the human race.
- Explain how critical thinking is an important element of the nursing process.
- List outstanding characteristics and benefits of the nursing process.

KEY TERMS

actual nursing
   diagnosis
assessment
care plan
client centered
collaboration
collaborative problem
critical thinking
decision making
diagnosis

evaluation
expected outcome
implementation
JCAHO
medical diagnosis
NANDA
nursing diagnosis
nursing intervention
nursing process
objective data

prioritize
problem solving
process
risk nursing diagnosis
strengths
subjective data
wellness nursing
   diagnosis

The **nursing process** is a step-by-step method of providing care to clients. While progressing through each step, the nurse uses a variety of skills that are purposeful and promote a systematic, orderly thought process. Discoveries are communicated to the client and other health care professionals, promoting continuity of client-centered care and giving structure to reality. The nursing process consists of five steps: assessment, diagnosis, planning and outcome identification, implementation, and evaluation.

This chapter provides a brief historical time line of the evolution of the nursing process, its outstanding characteristics, and an overview of each step. Chapter topics include discussion of the theoretical basis of the nursing process, the importance and necessity of critical thinking throughout all steps of the process, and the relationship between problem solving, decision making, and the nursing process.

WHAT IS A PROCESS?

The term **process** is defined as a series of planned actions or operations directed toward a particular result or goal. For example, ham stored in a smokehouse, an enclosed environment, is allowed to cook over slow-burning wood chips. The wood is selected specifically for the flavor it yields, like hickory or pecan. This aroma permeates the ham and, over time, cooks the meat, making it edible and palatable. The ham goes through a process called curing, the result of a series of planned actions or steps that are directed toward a particular goal.

NURSING PROCESS

The nursing process is defined as an _____, _____ method of planning and providing individualized care to clients. The nursing process is a tool promoting organization and utilization of the steps to achieve desired outcomes. The steps of the nursing process build upon each other, overlapping previous and subsequent steps. The nursing process may be used with clients throughout the life span and in any setting where care is provided to clients.

Unique Characteristics of the Nursing Process

The nursing process is a _____ and _____ method that is _____ based as well as _____ based. The nurse

TABLE 1:1 Timeline: Evolution of the Nursing Process

pre-1955	Before the nursing process evolved, the nurse provided care based on medical orders written by physicians. Care was initiated based on the caregiver's instinct to nurture. There were no clearly identifiable boundaries defined for nursing practice.
1955	The term nursing process was coined by Lydia Hall.
Late 1950's– early 1960's	Dorothy Johnson (1959), Ida Orlando (1961), and Ernestine Wiedenbach (1963) introduced a three-step nursing process model.
1966	Virginia Henderson identified the nursing process model as the same steps used in the scientific method: observing, measuring, gathering data, and analyzing the findings.
1967	A four-step model was proposed: assessment, planning, intervention, and evaluation.
1973	The use of the nursing process in clinical practice continued to gain additional accuracy and recognition when the American Nurses Association (ANA) published Standards of Clinical Nursing Practice (Table 1:2).
	Publication of Standards of Clinical Nursing Practice gave further legitimacy to the five phases or steps of the nursing process. Nursing educators and clinicians began to use the five-step nursing process model on a regular basis. National conferences were initiated in 1973, resulting in the beginning of the classification of nursing diagnoses. North American Nursing Diagnosis Association (NANDA) conferences have been held every two years since then for the purpose of identification, clarification, and refinement of nursing diagnoses.
1980	ANA published A Social Policy Statement, which provided guidelines (standards) for individual professional nurses to follow in practice.
1982	National Council Licensure Examination (NCLEX) was revised to include the nursing process concepts as a basis for organization.
1984	**Joint Commission on Accreditation of Healthcare Organizations (JCAHO)** launched requirements for accredited hospitals to use the nursing process as a means of documenting all phases of client care.
Current	Current: The nursing process is a five-step process: assessment, diagnosis, planning, implementation, and evaluation.

TABLE 1:2 Standards of Clinical Nursing Practice

Standards of Care

I. *Assessment*
The nurse collects client health data.

II. *Diagnosis*
The nurse analyzes the assessment data in determining diagnoses.

III. *Outcome Identification*
The nurse identifies expected outcomes individualized to the client.

IV. *Planning*
The nurse develops a plan of care that prescribes interventions to attain expected outcomes.

V. *Implementation*
The nurse implements the interventions identified in the care plan.

VI. *Evaluation*
The nurse evaluates the client's progress toward attainment of outcomes.

Standards of Professional Performance

I. *Quality of Care*
The nurse systematically evaluates the quality and effectiveness of nursing practice.

II. *Performance Appraisal*
The nurse evaluates his/her own nursing practice in relation to professional practice standards and relevant statutes and regulations.

III. *Education*
The nurse acquires and maintains current knowledge of nursing practice.

IV. *Collegiality*
The nurse contributes to the professional development of peers, colleagues, and others.

V. *Ethics*
The nurse's decisions and actions on behalf of clients are determined in an ethical manner.

VI. *Collaboration*
The nurse collaborates with the client, significant others, and health care providers in providing client care.

VII. *Research*
The nurse uses research findings in practice.

VIII. *Resource Utilization*
The nurse considers factors related to safety, effectiveness, and cost in planning and delivering client care.

From American Nurses Association. (1991). *Standards of clinical nursing practice.* Washington, DC: Author.

uses learned knowledge and comprehension of the human body to identify actual or potential health problems resulting from physical or psychological disease or disorders. Knowledge and understanding of fundamental philosophical views, such as Maslow's hierarchy of human needs (Figure 1:1), are essential to the practice of nursing and aid in identifying the expected response to illness or the client's sense of wellness.

The nursing process is _____, _____, and _____.
Using an orderly, step-by-step process, the client is evaluated, data are collected and

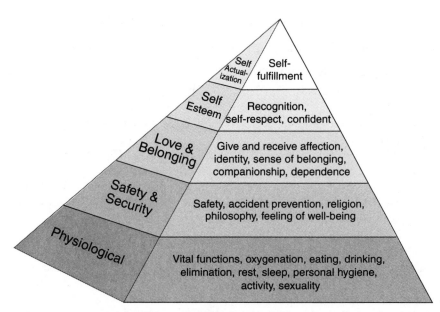

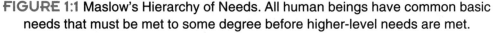

FIGURE 1:1 Maslow's Hierarchy of Needs. All human beings have common basic needs that must be met to some degree before higher-level needs are met.

analyzed, and a plan is formulated and set into motion. Client progress and response to treatment are continuously monitored and evaluated. The care plan is revised according to the changing needs of the client.

The nursing process is a map used to progress from point *a* to point *b*. The nursing process is a method used to _____ nursing activities. The ultimate goal is to _____ and _____ client wellness or to _____ the client's present state of health or sense of wellness.

The nursing process is recognized to be highly effective in promoting quality of care. A client entering the health care continuum receives a thorough, initial assessment. The needs and strengths of the client are identified. A **care plan** (documentation of the first, second, and third steps of the nursing process) is _____ and _____ to other health care professionals, so care is coordinated and ongoing. The client is continuously monitored for changing _____ and the plan is evaluated for appropriateness. Assessment and evaluation, which are constant, play a key role in realizing client needs, strengths, and response to treatment. Health care professionals _____, _____, and _____ the care plan, enhancing and promoting quality of care.

The nursing process serves as a _____, ensuring deliberate steps are taken which help avoid _____ and premature _____. It provides a _____ for which nurses use knowledge and skill to express human caring and to help clients meet their needs.

The nursing process is **client centered**, meaning care is focused on the client. The nurse organizes the care plan according to client _____ and/or

_____, rather than nursing _____. The client is encouraged to be an active participant in the nursing process, communicating needs and concerns and validating collected data. This gives the client a sense of control over his or her care.

Through the nursing process the nurse utilizes skills, such as _____, _____, and _____ skills.

Interpersonal Skills: _____

_____

_____

Technical Skills: _____

_____

Intellectual Skills: _____

_____

The nursing process promotes **collaboration** (communication with other disciplines to solve problems). As the client enters the health care system, individual professional responsibilities of the health care providers begin. Ongoing assessment of the client and response to care are monitored and recorded as physician orders and nursing interventions are carried out. Nursing professionals communicate necessary data through means of verbal reports and written documentation. Collaboration with the physician, nursing professionals, and other disciplines is often necessary to _____ care and _____ _____.

The nursing process is _____ _____. It is appropriate to institute and apply the nursing process with clients of any age. The nursing process may be incorporated at any point on the wellness-illness continuum in a variety of health-related settings including schools, hospitals, home health care facilities and clinics, and across specialties in hospital or acute care settings including intensive care, pediatrics, labor and delivery, medical surgical units, etc.

Use of the nursing process is beneficial to both the client and nurse. Examples of benefits include:

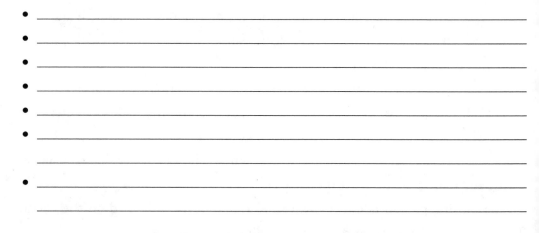

- _____
- _____
- _____
- _____
- _____
- _____
- _____

Each step of the nursing process is specific, in sequence, and interrelated.

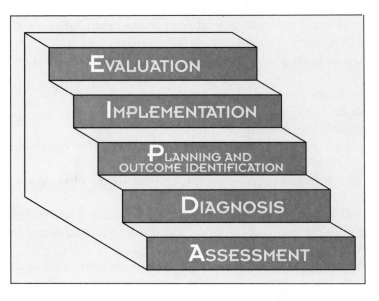

Step 1: Assessment

Assessment provides key information, compiled to form the client database. This phase involves several steps:

• Data collection: _____

_____

• Verification: _____

_____

• Organization: _____

• Interpretation: _____

• Documentation: _____

Two types of information are collected during the assessment step: objective and subjective data. Objective data are _____ or _____ information, accumulated through the physical exam, interview, or results of diagnostic examinations. Subjective data include the client's communicated _____, _____, _____, _____ or _____. A more detailed description of objective and subjective data can be found in chapter 2, "Assessment."

Step 2: Diagnosis

Diagnosis is the classification of a disease, condition, or human response based upon scientific evaluation of signs and symptoms, patient history, and diagnostic studies. Diagnosis involves analysis of collected data. After analysis, a list of nursing diagnoses or labels describing client problems or strengths is formulated. The nurse uses critical-thinking and decision-making skills in developing nursing diagnoses, a process facilitated by asking questions such as:

- What actual problems, if any, were identified during the assessment step?
- What are the possible causes of the problems?
- Is the client at risk for developing other problems; if so, what are the factors involved?
- Did the client indicate a desire to function at a higher level of wellness in a particular area?
- What are the client's strengths?
- What additional data might be needed to answer these questions?
- What are possible sources of data collection?
- Are there any identified problems that should be treated in collaboration with the physician?
- What data are pertinent to collect before contacting the physician?

During the diagnosis phase, existing problems requiring intervention from the nurse are identified. When the client demonstrates signs and symptoms, an actual problem exists. This type of problem is labeled as an actual nursing diagnosis. Potential problems a client may be at risk for developing are identified as well. Potential problems are labeled as risk nursing diagnoses. Potential or risk problems may be prevented by actions executed for the purpose of prevention.

Wellness nursing diagnoses may be identified and included in the plan of care, when the client has indicated a desire to attain a higher level of wellness in a particular area. The diagnostic label is preceded by the phrase *potential for enhanced*. For example, a client who is neither overweight nor underweight expresses a desire to gain more knowledge on how to reduce overall fat content of her diet for future health and prevention of disease. The nurse would identify the wellness nursing diagnosis of *Potential for Enhanced Nutrition*.

Strengths of the client are identified. These are areas of positive functioning used to support the care plan. For example, a client's family may be very supportive, giving encouragement and the desire to get well.

Potential complications requiring physician intervention that arise during treatment are identified and considered collaborative problems. Actions are initiated to resolve or reduce the risk of complication by implementing physician-prescribed orders in collaboration with nursing-prescribed interventions. The nurse primarily monitors for the onset and change in status of physiological complications. These usually are related to disease, trauma, treatments, medications, or diagnostic studies (Carpenito, 1997). Col-

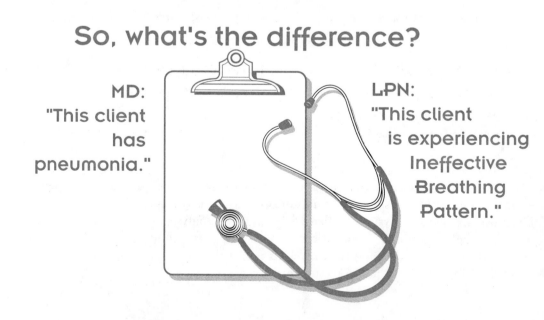

So, what's the difference?

MD:
"This client has pneumonia."

LPN:
"This client is experiencing Ineffective Breathing Pattern."

laborative problems are labeled as *Potential Complication (PC)* followed by the situation—for example, a client who has undergone surgical intervention, *PC: Hemorrhage* or a client who has experienced a myocardial infarction, *PC: Dysrhythmias*.

Clients receive both medical and nursing diagnoses. *Nursing diagnoses* should not be confused with *medical diagnoses*. Table 1:3 compares medical and nursing diagnoses.

Medical diagnoses are determined by the _____ indicating a disease or disorder identified or to be ruled out, e.g., pneumonia, renal failure, sepsis, or diabetes mellitus. Nursing diagnoses are problems identified and determined by the professional _____. *So, what makes the nursing diagnosis different?*

According to the North American Nursing Diagnosis Association (NANDA), a nursing diagnosis is a _____ _____ about individual, family, or community responses to actual or potential health problems/life processes. In 1980, the American Nurses Association defined nursing process as the diagnosis and treatment of _____ _____ to actual or potential health problems of disease and medical treatment.

The preceding statement means nurses are *not* responsible for diagnosing and ordering treatment for disorders such as cancer. Professional nurses diagnose and treat the client's _____ to cancer, such as inadequate nutrition, nausea, altered self-esteem, anxiety, and pain.

After data are analyzed and problems, risks, and strengths identified, a list of nursing diagnoses is formulated, then presented to the client for confirmation. If the client is unable to participate, family members may be able to assist in confirmation. Finally, the list of nursing diagnoses is recorded and the remainder of the client's care plan completed.

The client is continuously reassessed (Figure 1:2). Data are collected and documented during this process. As physician-prescribed treatments and nursing-prescribed interventions are carried out, the client demonstrates responses to the care provided. Response to treatment may involve improvement of health or the client's condition may worsen. Nursing diagnoses included in the care plan reflect the changing needs of the client.

TABLE 1:3 Comparison of Medical Diagnoses and Nursing Diagnosis

Medical Diagnoses	Nursing Diagnoses
• Determined by the physician	• Determined by nurses
• Indicate a disease or disorder identified or to be ruled out	• Indicate the client's response to illness, disease, or present state of health
• Remain constant until client recovers from disease or illness	• May change as the client responds to medical treatment, therapies, and nursing interventions
• Pneumonia	• Impaired gas exchange
• COPD exacerbation	• Ineffective breathing pattern
• Prostatitis	• Altered urinary elimination
• Acute renal failure	• Risk for impaired skin integrity

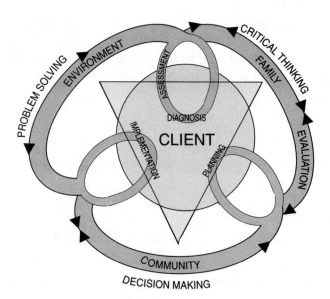

FIGURE 1:2 Nursing process is a method used to determine client needs. Assessment of the client and evaluation of the client and care plan are continuous. The nurse uses critical thinking, problem solving, and decision making throughout this process.

Step 3: Planning and Outcome Identification

Planning and outcome identification involve formulating and documenting the care plan. This phase of the nursing process organizes the proposed course of action for resolution of _____ problems and prevention of _____ problems. This task involves several steps:

- _____

- _____
  _____

- _____
  _____

Prioritizing problems means to decide which nursing diagnoses are most important and require attention first. Problems involving life-threatening situations are given the highest priority. An in-depth discussion of prioritizing problems can be found in chapter 4.

The absolute goal for any client is to achieve or maintain the greatest level of wellness possible. **Goals** are client centered, which means they focus on *behavior* of the client. Goals are broad statements describing the _____ or _____ _____ in the client's condition. An expected outcome is a particular expectation involving steps leading to the fulfillment of a goal, and therefore, resolution of the _____ of a problem. Goals and expected outcomes are used to evaluate the _____ of nursing interventions and the care plan.

Nursing interventions are activities executed to enable accomplishment of goals. They are nursing actions _____ and _____ with problem resolution in mind.

Step 4: Implementation

Implementation involves _____ of the nursing care plan. As planned interventions are _____, the nurse must continue to assess the client's condition before, during, and after each intervention is carried out. Reporting and documentation of collected data are important. Both positive and negative responses are reported and documented. _____ responses to treatment may require additional intervention. Chapter 5 provides an in-depth discussion of implementation. Implementation includes:

- _____
- _____
- _____

Step 5: Evaluation

During evaluation (appraisal of results), the nurse determines if client goals were _____, _____ _____, or _____ _____. If the goal has been met, the nurse must decide if or when nursing activities will cease. This decision will depend on the client's status. Can the client maintain the present level of wellness? If the goal has been partially met or not met, the nurse reactivates each step of the nursing process. Data must be collected to determine why the goal was not achieved and what modifications to the care plan are necessary. Refer to Table 1:4 for sample questions nurses ask to evaluate client care.

COGNITIVE SKILLS

When a client enters the health care system, nurses are involved in _____ _____. Care is planned for the client based on facts continuously col-

TABLE 1:4 Questions to Ask During Evaluation

- Are the interventions working?
- Is the current care plan helping the client make progress toward the goal?
- Has the client's status changed in any way? If so, is the plan still valid?
- Was the goal met or partially met?
- Was the goal realistic?
- Is there more that the health care team can do?
- Was the time frame too optimistic?
- Are goals and nursing interventions appropriate for the client?

lected and _____ throughout the nursing process. Skills vital to this process include _____ _____, _____ _____, and _____ _____.

Critical Thinking

Critical thinking is a purposeful _____ _____ incorporating various strategies in search for the meaning of data. Deliberate questions are asked in order to _____ and _____ evidence. Critical thinkers seek out explanations for what is happening. Examples of questions critical thinkers ask are found in Table 1:5.

Problem Solving

The nursing process is a **problem-solving** method. However, there is a difference between this method and the method used in solving daily problems. In both methods,

TABLE 1:5 Questions Critical Thinkers May Ask

Assessment	Have any data been omitted? Are there any data to be verified or validated that otherwise would lead to possible inaccuracies? Do subjective data complement and clarify objective data?
Diagnosis	What meaning is attached to collected data? What else could this mean? When clustering data, is there a pattern indicating specific problems? Is the client demonstrating signs or symptoms indicating they are at risk of developing future problems? Do the nursing diagnosis label and etiology accurately describe the problem? Did the client have adequate input into problem identification?
Planning and Outcome Identification	What are priority problems? Why are these problems priorities? What are the goals for the client? Are these goals realistic? What else might be accomplished? What interventions can assist the client in goal attainment? Is collaboration with other medical or health-related sources beneficial at this time? What other resources could benefit the client? Are planned interventions appropriate for the client, nurse, and facility?
Implementation	Has the client's condition changed since the last interaction? What is the client's current status? What interventions should be carried out first? Is the client demonstrating improvement in health status? Did the executed intervention result in the expected response? Why did the client respond in that manner?
Evaluation	Is the client progressing toward goal attainment? Are goals being met or only partially met? Is there more that can be done to alter the situation? Can the care plan be revised to be more effective? Was information accurate when initial data were collected? Was assessment thorough? Was each additional step of the nursing process followed through appropriately? Should additional data be collected? How can the plan be revised to best suit the client's needs?

Nursing Tip

Think about the whole clinical picture

If someone is having difficulty breathing or is in extreme pain . . .

Attend to this priority first!

information is gathered, problems are identified, specific problems are labeled, a plan is developed for solving the problem, the plan is put into action, and then, the results are evaluated. However, in solving daily problems, plans are frequently based on _____ data and sometimes on presumptions. This type of problem solving is more linear compared with the _____ and _____ nature of the nursing process. Nurses using the nursing process method of problem solving actively engage in taking deliberate steps and use critical thought to identify and solve problems.

Decision Making

Decision making, a skill used throughout the nursing process, is based on _____ and _____ based theories. Appropriate decision making and problem solving result from the nurse's ability to think critically, using perceptual and intellectual skills. This results in accurate problem identification, generating a reflective care plan and determining appropriate nursing interventions to aid in problem resolution. Interventions for each nursing diagnosis are selected based on _____ _____, *why* the intervention will work. An in-depth discussion of scientific rationales can be found in chapter 4, "Planning."

Key Concepts

- The nursing process is an organized, continuous, systematic method of planning, providing care, and problem solving. It is cyclic, ongoing, and dynamic.
- When a client enters the health care system, the nursing process begins. Use of the nursing process improves quality of care provided and promotes continuity of care.
- The nursing process consists of five interrelated steps: assessment, diagnosis, planning and outcome identification, implementation, and evaluation.
- Data collection utilizes a variety of sources and tools (*assessment*). Efforts are instituted to prevent omission or collection of inaccurate data.

- Data are organized and analyzed. Problems, potential problems, and strengths are identified and labeled (*diagnosis*).
- During the planning and outcome identification step, nursing diagnoses are prioritized. The professional nurse makes decisions on an appropriate course of action. The plan focuses on the client.
- Interventions are carried out (*implementation*).
- *Evaluation* of the plan and reassessment of the client are ongoing and continuous. The care plan is revised and updated when the client's needs change in response to medical treatment, therapies, and nursing interventions.
- *Care plan* revision may be necessary when the goal of treatment is partially met or not met.
- The care plan is developed, recorded, and placed in the client's chart, then communicated to other health care team members. This promotes ongoing continuity of care. The plan is reviewed for accuracy according to the policy of the facility and revised when needed.
- Nurses use perceptual and intellectual skills such as critical thinking, problem solving, and decision making.

APPLICATION EXAMPLE 1: PROBLEM SOLVING

It was Monday morning as Jay Brown performed his usual routine of getting ready for the trip across town to his office. He glanced at his watch as he finished eating breakfast; it was time to leave.

As Jay approached his automobile, he realized that one of the tires was flat. A nail was protruding from the center of the tire. Jay was forced to use his problem-solving capabilities, an everyday occurrence.

Step 1: Assessment

- Collection of data. Facts are gathered to describe and understand the actual or potential problem. In this case, it was obvious: flat tire, nail protruding from tire, unable to leave for work.

Step 2: Diagnosis

- Data are analyzed and problems identified, prioritized, and stated in a way that allows others to understand the problem.
- *Impaired Ability to Roll, Tire*. Related to: *Mechanical factors, decreased tire pressure*. As evidenced by: *Flat, deflated tire, nail protruding from tire*.

Step 3: Planning

- Questions are asked related to problem solving. What can be done about this problem? Is collaboration with other experts necessary or is this within my scope of practice/knowledge? What outcome should be achieved? What steps should be taken to resolve the situation?
- Jay knew his goal was to get to work on time, so he decided on a plan of action and determined priorities:
  1. First, call work to let them know he might be running late.
  2. Consult the owner's manual for instruction on how to change a tire.
  3. Check to make sure there is a spare tire, jack, and necessary tools.
  4. Review manual directions regarding the jack . . . etc., etc., until the step-by-step strategy is complete for changing the flat tire.

Step 4: Implementation

- Assess the client (in this case, the automobile tire) as interventions are executed. Carry out and perform the planned interventions.

Step 5: Evaluation

- As the steps are carried out, Jay takes a critical look at his progress. He evaluates the data, plan, overall goal, interventions, and whether he is truly making progress.

The process begins again, always assessing the situation, always evaluating the effectiveness of the plan. Jay's new tire was in place, holding air, and rolling easily. Even though the original problem seemed to be resolved, he knew the process was not over. He understood the problem-solving method was continuous and ongoing. As reassessment and evaluation occurred, new data were collected and a new problem identified—no spare tire for his automobile and the original tire was flat. So, planning began again to resolve the changing situation.

Basically, the preceding example shows how the nursing process can be used to problem solve: assessment, problem identification, decision making, planning, implementation, and evaluation.

APPLICATION EXAMPLE 2: PROBLEM SOLVING

June Brown, Jay's wife and a nursing student, was getting ready for a busy week. Marie, their preschooler, was to go to day care. Mrs. Brown went into the child's bedroom and realized Marie was not her usual active self.

Step 1: Assessment

- Immediately, Mrs. Brown began to gather data. Marie's face looked flushed. When Mrs. Brown touched her skin, it was very warm. Marie's temperature reading was 104.4°F. Mrs. Brown continued to assess her child for other signs of illness. Numerous questions went through her mind as she performed a physical assessment. When all the data were gathered, she began to sort them out.

Step 2: Diagnosis

- One obvious problem was identified. Mrs. Brown labeled the problem using an approved nursing diagnosis which accurately defines the observed problem. This is not a *medical* diagnosis; nurses do not have that responsibility.
- Mrs. Brown was unsure of Marie's medical illness; however, she was able to identify one response to her illness: *Hyperthermia. Related to (R/T): Illness. As evidenced by (AEB):* Increase in body temperature above normal range, temperature 104.4°F, flushed skin, skin warm to touch.

Step 3: Planning

- June Brown thought about the preceding problem statement and what could be done. Her primary goal/outcome was to reduce the child's fever. During this phase of planning, Mrs. Brown identified priority problems, established goals, and determined interventions. (If she were in clinical, she would have reviewed physician orders.)

Goal/Outcome Identification: Marie will experience a reduced body temperature within forty-five minutes of intervention.

Interventions were determined:

1. Administer Tylenol (decide on amount to administer and route).
2. Provide cool liquids by mouth, offer popsicle, juice.
3. For temperature that continues to rise higher than 104.6°F, provide tepid sponge bath, prevent chilling.
4. Reevaluate temperature status within forty-five minutes after any intervention.
5. Consult pediatrician as needed.

Step 4: Implementation

- Execute the plan. Mrs. Brown prepared to give Marie Tylenol. Upon entering the bedroom, she continued to assess and monitor her young daughter, looking for other signs and symptoms that were new or possibly missed. Just prior to receiving the Tylenol, Marie began to vomit (problem identified). Quickly, June began to evaluate her plan of care. She determined the original plan was appropriate, however, it did need a slight revision. She decided to administer a Tylenol suppository instead of the liquid by mouth.

Step 5: Evaluation

- Did the plan work? Was the goal achieved? Was Marie's body temperature decreased within forty-five minutes and has she remained afebrile (without fever)? Was the goal partially achieved, or not at all? Have other problems been identified? Are there changes to make in the care plan to make it more effective?

During the ongoing assessment and evaluation, a new problem, *vomiting*, was identified. This must be added to the problem list. What physiological effect could this have on the body? If it were long lasting, it would affect *nutrition* and/or *fluid volume*. The appropriate nursing diagnoses for these risk problems are as follows: *Risk for Altered Nutrition: Less than Body Requirements* and *Risk for Fluid Volume Deficit*. The term *risk* is used because the child could potentially develop the problems, although they have not yet occurred.

STUDENT PRACTICE: PROBLEM SOLVING USING THE NURSING PROCESS
Instructions

Read the scenario below and provide answers to the following:

a. List all problem(s).
b. From the problem list, identify one priority nursing diagnosis.
c. Locate and write the definition of the nursing diagnosis.
d. What are *related to* and *as evidenced by* criteria?

1. Jason Jefferson, twenty-seven years old, arrived at the clinic around 11:30 A.M. complaining of excruciating, continuous pain in his jaw. He said he had only been in town for a week and had not found a dentist. His tooth had been hurting for two days. During assessment of the client's mouth (oral mucosa), the nurse observed Mr. Jefferson's gums were red and swollen. He had several unfilled cavities (dental caries) and poor dental hygiene.

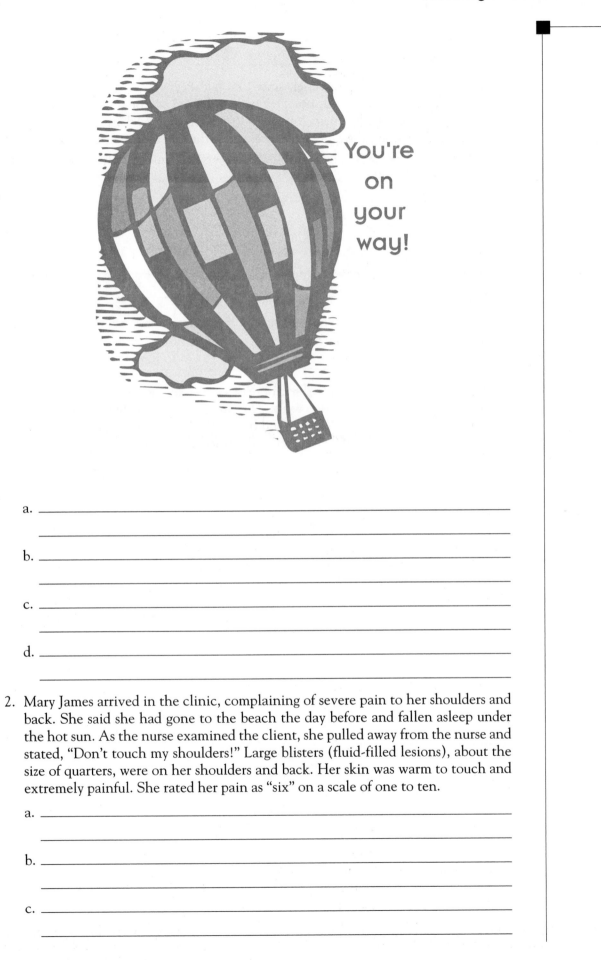

You're
on
your
way!

a. _____

_____

b. _____

_____

c. _____

_____

d. _____

_____

2. Mary James arrived in the clinic, complaining of severe pain to her shoulders and back. She said she had gone to the beach the day before and fallen asleep under the hot sun. As the nurse examined the client, she pulled away from the nurse and stated, "Don't touch my shoulders!" Large blisters (fluid-filled lesions), about the size of quarters, were on her shoulders and back. Her skin was warm to touch and extremely painful. She rated her pain as "six" on a scale of one to ten.

a. _____

_____

b. _____

_____

c. _____

_____

d. _____

_____

3. Terrence McPherson, a rancher, stated he had been walking in his pasture last week, stepped into a gopher hole, tripped, and fell down on a jagged, sharp metal object. He sustained a deep, two-inch (five-centimeter) laceration on his left forearm. The wound was not bleeding at the time of examination; however, the tissue around the wound was reddened and swollen. The nurse observed clear fluid draining from the wound.

a. _____

_____

b. _____

_____

c. _____

_____

d. _____

_____

4. Marjorie Taylor was diagnosed with breast cancer six months ago. Her physician performed a left radical mastectomy. The surgical site is healed; however, she experiences swelling in her left arm and hand. She states, "Sometimes my arm is so heavy, I can hardly lift it." Her doctor identifies this as lymphedema.

a. _____

_____

b. _____

_____

c. _____

_____

d. _____

_____

Assessment

"What you want are facts, not opinions. . . . The most important practical lesson that can be given to nurses is to teach them what to observe—how to observe. . . .

For it may safely be said, not that the habit of ready and correct observation will by itself make us useful nurses, but that without it we shall be useless with all our devotion.

But if you cannot get in the habit of observation one way or the other, you had better give up being a nurse, for it is not your calling, however kind and anxious you may be.

It [observation] is not for the sake of piling up miscellaneous information or curious facts, but for the sake of saving life and increasing health and comfort."

Florence Nightingale

OBJECTIVES

Upon completion of this chapter, the student should be able to:

- Identify and describe the components of assessment.
- Differentiate between objective and subjective data.
- Describe the concept of data collection and discuss methods and sources involved in data collection.
- Discuss the importance of establishing a baseline database for comparison of future data.
- Discuss the unique characteristics of the assessment step.
- Identify modes of communication.
- Describe the purpose of therapeutic communication.
- Describe interview preparation and conducting the interview.
- Discuss the three phases of an interview.

KEY TERMS

analyze	inspection	percussion
assessment	interpret	social communication
auscultation	interview	subjective data
baseline data	introduction phase	therapeutic
closed question	objective data	communication
closure	observation	validation
data clustering	open-ended question	verification
holistic	palpation	working phase

ASSESSMENT: STEP 1 OF THE NURSING PROCESS

Assessment is the first step in the nursing process. It involves the act of gathering _____ about the health status of a client (individual, resident, group of individuals). The information is _____ using a systematic approach, then _____, _____, _____, and _____ to ensure its accuracy. Finally, data are documented. The care plan is developed from assessment activities, such as the client interview and physical assessment.

Initial data collected become the _____ of the client database and are termed baseline data. Thorough and accurate data collection is an important element in planning effective client care. The professional nurse uses deliberate thought processes, judgment, and problem-solving skills as data are _____, _____, _____, _____, and _____.

Data accumulated after the initial assessment are frequently *compared* to baseline data to determine the client's progress or improvement or to discover trends reflecting deterioration of the client's health status.

Example: Mr. Gomez, a fifty-eight-year-old Hispanic male, has been seen for his annual physical exam consecutively over the last several years. His first visit at the clinic was six years ago. At that time, baseline data were collected, including physical assessment, blood chemistry, and vital signs, of which all were within the normal range: blood pressure 128/82, pulse eighty-four, respirations eighteen. Today, Mr. Gomez's blood pressure measurement was 154/96. This value was compared to the previous blood pressure readings beginning with the initial baseline values and those obtained subsequently. The nurse discovered Mr. Gomez's blood pressure had progressively elevated over the years. The nurse brought this fact to the physician's attention. Further assessment, evaluation, and medical treatment will focus on minimizing and preventing the adverse effects of hypertension.

Nursing Tip

The care plan is developed, based on data gathered from the assessment.

Characteristics of Assessment

Assessment is the _____ step; however, it is systematic, ongoing, and continuous. Assessment is the process of collecting data (information) to identify _____ or _____ health problems and strengths of the client. The data provides a sense of the client's _____ _____ _____. Data collection may include physical, psychological, social, cultural, spiritual, and cognitive areas, as well as developmental level, economic status, functional abilities, and lifestyle, depending on the tool used during data collection.

Data are gathered during an _____, physical _____, and review of diagnostic studies. Information is analyzed and validated, and facts are clustered into groups of information to identify patterns of health or illness. Assessment data are accessible to other health care team members through _____ and _____.

DATA COLLECTION

Data collection begins when the client _____ the health care system. The nurse may begin collection prior to initial contact with the client through review of medical records and history. Collection continues during _____, _____, and _____. Data collection continues as long as there is a need for health care.

> ### Nursing Tip
>
> *Assessment = data collection, verification, organization, interpretation, and documentation.*

Types of Data

Data may be separated into two categories, subjective and objective data. Subjective data, also known as **symptoms**, are statements, feelings, perceptions, or concerns communicated by a client. For example, "I'm tired" or "I'm having pain" or "I feel so afraid." Objective data, also referred to as **signs**, can be observed, measured, or felt by someone other than the person experiencing them. Table 2:1 compares subjective and objective data.

TABLE 2:1 Subjective and Objective Data

Subjective	Objective
• What the person states, e.g., "I'm sad."	• Things that are observable and measurable by the examiner
• These are feelings and perceptions.	• Blood pressure of 110/70
• "I feel sick to my stomach."	• Rash on right arm
• "I wish I were home."	• Ambulates with a cane
• "I have a burning pain in my side."	• Ate 100% of breakfast
• "I feel like nobody likes me."	• 425 mL clear urine
• "My heart feels like it's racing."	

The author recommends that, as novice nurses, students separate collected data into subjective and objective data. Each category will _____ and _____ the other.

Example:
- Subjective data (what the subject states): "I feel like my heart is racing"
- Objective data: Pulse 150 beats per minute, regular, strong

> **Nursing Tip**
>
> *S—S: Subjective data are stated*
> *O—O: Objective data are observable*

Objective data _____ the subjective data. What the nurse observes and measures _____ what the client is feeling and experiencing. However, this may not always be true. There may be times when objective data will conflict or seem different from what the client is stating.

Example:
- Subjective data: Client states, "I can breathe fine"
- Objective data: Color pale, becomes easily short of breath with minimal exertion, respirations twenty-six per minute

In cases where data appear to conflict, the nurse should _____ the situation and gather all pertinent data to _____ the problem.

Sources of Data

Gathering data should involve every possible source. However, the client should be the _____ _____ of information, when possible. Family or

> **Nursing Tip**
>
> *Just state the facts. Do not state opinions and do not jump to conclusions. See Table 2:2.*

significant others may provide useful or additional information about the client. Data may be obtained from _____ _____, _____ _____, and verbal or written _____. Other members of the health care team working with the client may provide valuable information. Additional sources include _____ _____ (past and present) and relevant _____, for example, accepted standards (which indicate normal functioning, such as the accepted range of a normal pulse rate).

Data Collection Tools

The assessment database should include all aspects of the client's health status. Assessment tools are designed to help nurses _____ what data to collect and to _____ the information obtained. Health care facilities develop

TABLE 2:2 Subjective and Objective Data Versus Opinions and Conclusions

Subjective Data	Opinion or Conclusion
• "Don't let anyone else in my room."	• Client is angry or hostile.
• "I don't want to have that test."	• Client is anxious.
• "Get this tube out of my nose. It's killing me."	• Client is experiencing pain.
• "How do I get back to my room?"	• Client is disoriented.
• "Why hasn't the doctor seen me today?"	• Client is worried.

Objective Data	Opinion or Conclusion
• Dressed and shaved this morning	• Able to attend to ADLs (activities of daily living)
• Unsteady on feet when ambulating	• Client is intoxicated.
• Hands tremble	• Client is afraid or anxious.
• Heart rate 106 beats per minute	• Client is afraid or exercising.
• Client is lying in dark room during the day.	• Client is depressed or sad.
• Voided 300 mL amber urine	• Urine output is adequate.
• Able to change dressing to wound	• Understands sterile technique.
• Requests pain medication every two hours	• Client is addicted.

preprinted documents, which serve as a guide for collecting and recording necessary information. Appendix B contains examples of data collection tools. Most health care facilities use assessment tools based on nursing models considered holistic. This term means:

_____.

_____

_____

Otherwise, important information relating to how the client lives his or her daily life may be omitted or missed.

Some tools are organized based on problems commonly encountered on a particular nursing unit. For example, pediatric and geriatric data collection tools have additional questions pertaining to these age groups. Any format is acceptable, as long as it is thorough and comprehensive and considers the client's developmental age.

> **Nursing Tip**
>
> *Assessment is a key step in the nursing process.*

Methods of Data Collection

The nurse collects data through the following methods: _____, _____, and physical _____.

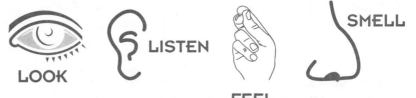

Use your senses of observation

LOOK   LISTEN   FEEL   SMELL

Note the client's overall general appearance - Thin?
Obese? Well-groomed? Does the client look their stated age?

Note body language/posture. How are they sitting?
Are they withdrawing? Are they makeing eye contact?
Observe the client's facial expressions.

Be aware of your method of interaction. Are you too close?
Too far away? Remember cultural differences.

FIGURE 2:1

Observation

The nurse uses observation (the skill of watching thoughtfully and deliberately) to discern the client's overall _____ and _____. Observations should include _____ and _____ responses, _____ of the client, and _____ with family or the nurse, as well as _____ or _____ characteristics, some of which may help or hinder data collection (Figure 2:1). These observations and others are made during initial and subsequent interactions with the client. Table 2:3 provides a checklist to aid in observation techniques.

The ability to communicate is central to the practice of nursing. It is a fundamental element in establishing a restorative nurse-client relationship. Communication includes the ability to appropriately _____, _____, and

TABLE 2:3 Aids to Observation

- Use your senses _____
- Note the client's general appearance _____
  _____
- Note body language _____
  _____
- Be aware of own interaction patterns _____
  Remember cultural differences relating to behavior.

TABLE 2:4 Overcoming Cultural Communication Barriers

- When the client and nurse speak different languages, obtain an interpreter to facilitate communication.
- Even though a client of a different culture and a nurse may speak the same language, verify the client's understanding of the exchange. Words may have different meanings to different people.
- Nonverbal communication, such as facial expression, posture, gestures, lack of eye contact, and use of silence are communication variances often misinterpreted.
- Consider social and family relationships, religion, language, food, and cultural view of health or illness when working with clients from differing cultures.
- Maintain a nonjudgmental attitude.
- Recognize biases.

_____ thoughts, feelings, and facts. In addition, nurses must be aware of cultural differences and variances related to communication. When cultural variances exist, inaccurate interpretation of communication may occur. Table 2:4 describes ways of overcoming possible cultural communication barriers.

Interview

An interview is a communication exchange between the client and nurse. This exchange has a _____ _____, which is to collect information about the client. Discoveries relating to the client's present and past health status allow the nurse to make determinations and decisions about health needs. Nurses use knowledge of communication to discerningly obtain _____ and _____. This information is gathered through conversation and observations during the structured interview. Developing interviewing skills takes time and practice.

There are different types of communication: _____ and _____. For the purpose of data collection, the nurse uses therapeutic communication. This interaction results in conversations with a client which are neither idle nor meaningless, but purposeful, goal-directed, focused on the client, and planned. Social communication is casual conversation, spontaneous and with no planned agenda.

Interview Preparation

Preparation and planning are key to effective interviewing. Suggestions for preparation include reviewing medical records, reviewing current admission documentation of past or present client care, and researching present and past medical diagnoses. In addition, forethought should be given to _____ for overcoming potential communication barriers which might impede successful data collection during the interview process. Table 2:5 identifies common barriers to therapeutic interaction.

TABLE 2:5 Barriers to Therapeutic Interaction

Barrier	Example
• Language differences	• Difficulty navigating through health care system • Prevents evaluation of client's response to nursing interventions
• Sociocultural differences	• Use of language may differ from nurse. Interpretation of words may be different
• Gender	• Communication can vary between men and women.
• Health status	• The disoriented or confused client is unable to reliably communicate. • Alterations in sensory or perceptual function, such as impairment or loss of vision, hearing, or sense of touch, affect the ability to send or receive communication messages. • Moderate to severe pain or discomfort and other health-related difficulties, such as dyspnea, may impair communication.
• Developmental level	• May require a different approach, different language, or different terminology in order for a client (for example, a child) to understand.
• Knowledge differences	• Client and family may have varying levels of education. Listen to conversations and vocabulary chosen. Consider the client's mental capabilities.
• Emotional distance	• Therapeutic communication involves establishing a caring, empathetic relationship with the client. Emotional distance refers to a barrier existing between the client and nurse which prevents effective therapeutic communication. Examples include a client in respiratory isolation or a comatose or confused client.
• Emotions	• Fear, anxiety, and depression are examples of emotions that prevent therapeutic communication.
• Daydreaming	• Allowing one's mind to wander instead of being an active listener may lead to missing the point of the message. Nurses must be attentive, alert, and focused on the conversation.

Conducting the Interview

The interview most often occurs at the beginning of the nurse-client relationship. The nurse may institute various techniques in an effort to build rapport with the client (Figure 2:2). Rapport promotes positive interactions between the health care team and client.

Tips to help you establish rapport with the client

MAINTAIN EYE CONTACT

1. Interview in a private setting - environment should be quiet, private. Turn down the TV. Close the room door.

2. When addressing the client, use appropriate title. Introduce yourself.

3. State the purpose of the exchange/interview. Explain why you will be asking questions.

4. Maintain eye contact - do not stare, but be attentive.

5. Do not rush through the data collection tool. Use a caring, interested manner, clarifying and investigating, when appropriate.

FIGURE 2:2

Techniques that advocate productive, therapeutic communication include:

_____

_____

_____

Controlling the environment, making it more conducive for the interview, is an important part of preparation. This includes providing _____, allowing adequate _____ for answering questions, maintaining a comfortable room temperature, reducing environmental _____ levels, and eliminating or decreasing _____, if possible.

There are three phases to an interview: introduction, working, and closure. During the introduction phase of the interview, goals for the interaction are stated. Both the purpose and use of collected data should be discussed. For example, the nurse might begin by stating, "I need to ask you a few questions about your health, so I can better plan for your care." Inform the client how long the interview will last.

The working phase of the interview focuses on the details of data collection. The assessment interview may consist of collecting comprehensive data, for example, a detailed past medical history, as well as a thorough physical examination. An assessment interview may also be focused on a specific area, such as data collection regarding pain description. Specific data collection tool formats are used during the assessment interview and will aid in data organization. The tool will depend on the type of information to be collected and the model accepted and used by the facility.

Data collection is facilitated by various communication techniques. During the interview, nurses ask questions to elicit a particular response. How questions are asked will determine client responses (Figure 2:3). Open-ended questions are stated in a manner that encourages the client to _____ about a particular concern or

Interviewing Techniques

1. Make sure your questions are relevant to the reason the client is seeking health care.

2. Use correct terminology - remember age appropriate terms and use terms the client can understand. Do not talk down to the client.

3. Use open-ended questions and comments, reflection, summarize, restate...communication techniques.

4. Use an organized, systematic assessment tool.

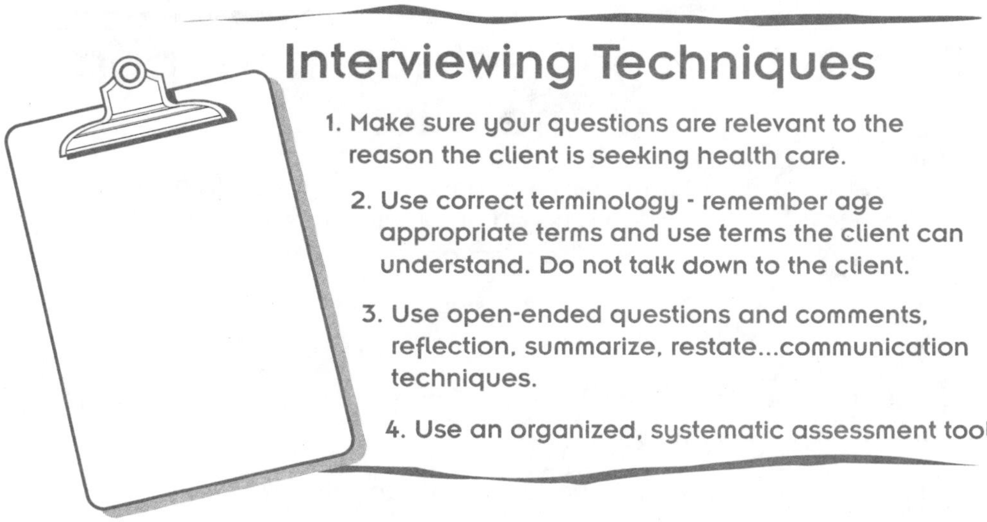

FIGURE 2:3

problem. For example, "What types of food do you usually eat during a twenty-four-hour period?" or "What led to your coming here today?" Each of these questions encourages the client to respond with information. Closed questions can be answered with brief _____ answers. This type of questioning may be appropriate in certain situations, for example, in an emergency: "Did she respond to you when you entered her room?" or "How many pounds has she lost over the last month?" Additional techniques that promote communication during an interview or therapeutic nurse-client communication can be found in Table 2:6 and Figure 2:4.

TABLE 2:6 Therapeutic Communication Techniques

Technique	Example
Offering self	Being present and available for client. Example: "Let's talk for a while"
Using silence	Remain quiet, allow the client time to reflect on the conversation and collect her thoughts.
Use of open-ended comments	Promotes client response. Example: "Yes, go on . . ." or "You were saying . . ."
Reflection	Repeating the last words spoken by the client. Example: The client says, "I feel so frustrated!" and the nurse says, "Frustrated?" This prompts the client to provide further explanation.
Giving a general lead	Promotes direction to the interaction. Example: "Tell me more about the . . ."
Focusing	The nurse focuses on the topic that may require clarification, such as, "You mentioned that you had . . ."
Observing	Calling attention to a specific behavior, such as, "You seem to be in pain"

Promoting a Successful Interview

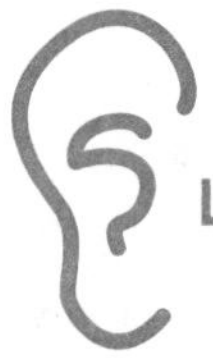

LISTEN!

1. Listen actively! Convey acceptance - make eye contact, nod your head to show interest. Be attentive - concentrate on the client's words.

2. Allow client/family member to finish sentences/thoughts - don't interrupt.

3. Be patient - allow time for client to answer or respond.

4. When appropriate, summarize and restate.

FIGURE 2:4

Bringing Closure to the Interview

The nurse should indicate in some manner that the interview session is coming to an end. For example, the nurse could state that most of the information has been collected and only a few more facts are necessary. During closure, the nurse allows the client to present _____ _____ _____ and then _____ overall information that has been covered or accomplished. The nurse determines if additional sessions will be necessary for further exploration and, if so, plans are made with the client.

Physical Examination

The purpose of a physical examination is to _____ _____ regarding the client's present health status and to establish a _____ physical assessment. _____ observations can be made which may indicate deviations from normal. _____ and _____ of any subjective complaints may be obtained.

Nursing Tip

- *Always promote communication while assessing.*
- *Ask questions and then allow time for response.*
- *Do not rely on memory. Write it down.*
- *Choose a method for organizing your assessment, e.g., head to toe, body systems.*

During a physical examination the nurse uses various techniques to collect data. Initial physical data collected, known as baseline data, are documented and used for comparison and evaluation of the client's status at a given point in time.

Physical Examination Techniques

Physical assessment techniques include *inspection, auscultation, palpation,* and *percussion.* A brief description of each technique follows.

Inspection is a systematic process of _____ that includes vision. Through sight, the nurse observes skin color and condition, notes drainage, the effort to breathe, and respiratory pattern. Inspection includes noting one's body posture, gait, ability to use extremities, and facial expressions or observing the client's ability to carry out activities of daily living (ADLs).

Lighting: _____

Privacy: _____

Communicate: _____

Auscultation is the technique of _____ for sounds within the body, usually with a stethoscope. Areas most often auscultated include lungs, heart, abdomen, and blood vessels.

Palpation is an assessment technique involving use of _____ or pressing on the external surface of the body with the fingers. Palpation is used to assess _____, _____, _____, organ _____ and _____, vibrations and pulsations, swelling, masses, and tenderness. Examples of uses of palpation include:

• Touch: _____

• Pressure: _____

• Deep palpation: _____

Percussion is the technique involving direct or indirect _____ of a specific body surface to glean information about internal organs beneath the body surface. The health care provider may use _____, _____, or percussion _____ to elicit various tones indicating presence or absence of fluid or air, masses, consolidation, tenderness, and normal or abnormal reflexes.

DATA VERIFICATION AND VALIDATION

After all data are gathered, information is verified (confirmed or proved) and validated (determined to be fact) to ensure accuracy. Data are reviewed for _____, _____ or possible _____. For example, a confused client is admitted to the medical surgical unit, stating that he has no family. However, you were told that the person who brought him in was his wife. In another example, a client may state that he ambulates without difficulty and without the use of assistive devices. The client's wife states he uses a cane. The nurse observes the

Nursing Tip

Identify problems by asking the following questions:

1. Has the client experienced any change in his or her usual functional pattern?

2. Has the client demonstrated any indication of abnormal functioning of a body system?

3. Has the client demonstrated deviation from normal range when compared to standards?

client ambulating with an unsteady gait. In each case, the nurse would need to consider possible reasons for the discrepancy and collect more information before forming conclusions and planning care.

INTERPRETATION AND ORGANIZATION OF DATA

Data which have been collected, verified, and validated for accuracy are now ready to be analyzed (processing information to reach a conclusion) and interpreted (determining the meaning and significance). For this process, the nurse assigns meaning to collected data and groups data into clusters. Data are compared against standards such as normal health patterns, normal vital signs, lab values, basic food groups, or normal growth and development. Interpreting and analyzing data help identify missing _____ or _____. Once these are identified, it would be necessary to gather more data.

Data clustering is used to determine the _____ of facts, to find _____, and to determine if further data is needed.

Example:

Sharon O'Reilly, a thirty-eight-year-old female, was diagnosed with rheumatoid arthritis at the age of twenty. She states that at first, joints in her wrists and fingers were stiff and sometimes painfully swollen, but would resolve without intervention. She thought the symptoms were related to her active lifestyle. Over time, other joints became involved. Bilateral knees, right ankle, and right hand and fingers are painful, reddened, and edematous. She states she has difficulty performing even the simplest activities, such as brushing her hair or teeth or ambulating to the bathroom. The client was observed having difficulty brushing her hair and putting on her gown. She experiences almost constant pain, which she rates as "six" on a scale of one to ten. The nurse observes Ms. O'Reilly's face is masked with pain. She guards her knees, so that no one touches them. She asked for her walker as she attempted to ambulate to a chair. The nurse observes that she walks with a limp. She states she began to use a walker "about a year ago."

Subjective and Objective Data:

Subjective Data

- States she has difficulty performing activities
- States she is in almost constant pain
- Rates pain as "six" on scale of one to ten
- States she has used a walker for about a year

Objective Data

- Bilateral knees, right ankle, right hand and fingers reddened, edematous
- Facial mask of pain
- Guarding behavior
- Difficulty brushing hair and dressing
- Walks with a limp
- Observed difficulty ambulating
- Uses a walker to ambulate

Data Clustering:

Pain

- States bilateral knees, right ankle, right hand and fingers are painful
- Rates pain as "six" on scale of one to ten
- Facial mask of pain
- Guarding behavior

Self-Care

- States she has difficulty carrying out activities of daily living
- Observed difficulty dressing self and brushing hair

Mobility

- Uses a walker
- Has difficulty ambulating
- Walks with a limp

Data clustering _____ data, helps determine the _____ of subjective and objective data, and helps find _____ in the data. Data clustering provides _____ that specific problems exist and should be included in the care plan. In Sharon O'Reilly's case scenario, data are first separated into subjective and objective data, then clustered to determine patterns.

The clustered data support the fact that problems exist: *Chronic Pain, Impaired Physical Mobility,* and *Self-Care Deficit.* All subjective and objective data supporting the nursing diagnosis of pain are clustered together, confirming that the problem exists and interventions are necessary.

DOCUMENTING ASSESSMENT DATA

Documentation of data collected during the assessment is essential. Documentation is the process of preparing a record that reflects the assessment data and describes the client's present health status. When documenting this information, the nurse communicates with others involved in the client's care. This is necessary to provide quality care.

Various formats are utilized for documentation, depending on the agency. Data may be documented using narrative notations, checklists, a combination of the two, or specialty formats. Chapter 5 discusses and describes different types of documentation. Appendix B includes examples of assessment data collection tools and documentation forms.

Key Concepts

- Assessment is the first step in the nursing process. Information is gathered through an interview, physical examination, and review of diagnostic tests. These data reveal a sense of the overall health status of the client.
- Assessment is ongoing throughout the nursing process sequence.

- During assessment data are collected, organized, interpreted, verified, validated, and then documented.
- The care plan is developed from and based on data collected during initial and on-going assessment.
- Two types of data are collected: subjective and objective. Generally, each category will complement and clarify the other.
- The client should be the primary source of information. When this is not possible, family or significant others may provide useful or additional information about the client.
- Data sources include the client, nursing records, medical records, verbal and written consultations, diagnostic results, and relevant literature.
- Methods of data collection include observation, interview, and physical examination.
- Collected data should be verified and validated to ensure accuracy. Data should be reviewed for omissions and incongruities. If these are discovered, possible reasons for the discrepancy or inaccuracy should be identified and corrected.
- Clustering helps to organize data and determine the *relatedness* of subjective and objective information. Clustering also aids in finding patterns. This technique provides confirmation that an identified problem exists and should be included in the care plan.

STUDENT PRACTICE: DEVELOPING COMMUNICATION AND DATA COLLECTION
Instructions

Provide responses to the following:

1. Review and write characteristics of therapeutic communication.
2. Discuss communication skills that promote therapeutic communication.
3. Discuss the role of observation in data collection.
4. To support an understanding of the interview exchange, research the key elements of a successful interview.

STUDENT PRACTICE: DEVELOPING OPEN-ENDED QUESTIONS
Instructions

Change the following "closed" questions to open-ended questions or comments to promote therapeutic communication.

1. "Are you feeling better?"

_____

_____

2. "Did you like the dinner?"

_____

_____

3. "Are you in pain?"

_____

_____

4. "Do you understand what the doctor told you about the surgery?"

_____

_____

5. "Do you understand the doctor's instructions?"

_____

_____

STUDENT PRACTICE: DEVELOPING THERAPEUTIC COMMUNICATION TECHNIQUES
Instructions

Write a therapeutic communication techniques comment to promote therapeutic communication. You may refer to necessary resources.

1. Using reflection: Client makes the comment "Nothing ever goes right for me."

_____

_____

2. Using observation: Client is extremely quiet, talking softly.

_____

_____

3. Using open-ended comments: Client states, "They told me I had cancer just . . ."

_____

_____

4. Using restating: Client states, "I felt full even before I started eating."

_____

_____

5. Using focusing: The client goes into a long explanation about the problems he has experienced since he fell and broke his hip.

_____

_____

STUDENT PRACTICE: IDENTIFYING OBJECTIVE AND SUBJECTIVE DATA
Instructions

Underline _abnormal_ data discovered in the situations below. List subjective and objective data.

Situation: John Branson, a sixty-five-year-old African American male, was admitted into the hospital on your unit yesterday with shortness of breath. He quickly states, "I feel like I can't breathe." When he speaks, he becomes short of breath. He states that over the past few months, he has had to sleep propped on three pillows, and says, "I feel like I'm smothering if I don't." Mr. Branson has a medical history of congestive heart failure, which was diagnosed two years ago. Supplemental oxygen is in place, two liters via nasal cannula. Pulse oximeter reads ninety-four percent saturation. Physical assessment data include vital signs, blood pressure 144/92, pulse rate ninety-two per minute; coarse rales are auscultated in the anterior, bilateral bases of the lungs; respirations are slightly labored and increased, twenty-six per minute. He coughs as he takes a deep breath, however, it is nonproductive. He is afebrile; two-plus pitting edema to bilateral ankles and feet; pedal pulses are palpable, however, diminished; radial pulses strong and equal; capillary refill is sluggish, greater than three seconds.

1. List abnormal subjective data in the case history above.

_____

_____

_____

2. List abnormal objective data in the case history above.

_____

_____

_____

_____

Situation: Sandra Weston, a thirty-six-year-old Caucasian female, was admitted into the hospital with a medical diagnosis of cholecystitis (gallbladder disease). She states she is having severe pain, rated as "eight" on a scale of one to ten. She has been receiving an analgesic for pain every four hours as needed. The nurse giving the report states Ms. Weston has had numerous bouts of vomiting and is unable to eat or drink fluids. The physician was contacted, but has not returned the call. Ms. Weston has an IV for hydration in her right forearm. The client is scheduled for surgery in the morning. The client's vital signs are: blood pressure 136/88, pulse 106, respiration twenty-four, temperature 99.2°F. Her weight and height are 172 pounds and five feet three inches. She states that foods high in fat cause her to have pain in her stomach.

1. List abnormal subjective data in the case history above.

_____

_____

_____

_____

2. List abnormal objective data in the case history above.

_____

_____

_____

_____

Diagnosis

"Can such an illness be unaccompanied with suffering? Will any care prevent such a patient from suffering this or that?—I humbly say, I do not know. But when you have done away with all that pain and suffering, which in patients are the symptoms not of their disease, but of the absence of one or all of the above-mentioned essentials to the success of Nature's reparative processes, we shall then know what are the symptoms of and the sufferings inseparable from the disease.

With the sick, pain gives warning of the injury.

Irresolution is what all patients most dread. Rather than meet this in others, they will collect all their data, and make up their minds for themselves.

. . . the power of forming any correct opinion as to the result must entirely depend upon an enquiry [sic] into all the conditions in which the patient lives.

. . . a person of no scientific knowledge whatever but of observation and experience in these kinds of conditions, will be able to arrive at a much truer guess as to the probable duration of life of members of a family or inmates of a house, than most scientific physicians to whom the same persons are brought to have their pulse felt; no enquiry being made into their conditions."

Florence Nightingale

OBJECTIVES

Upon completion of this chapter, the student should be able to:

- Identify characteristics of nursing diagnoses.
- Identify and discuss differences between medical and nursing diagnoses.
- Describe the different types of nursing diagnoses.
- List components of actual and risk nursing diagnoses.
- Describe the process of developing a nursing diagnosis.

KEY TERMS

actual nursing
  diagnosis
defining
  characteristics

diagnosis
etiology
medical diagnosis
nursing diagnosis

problem
problem statement
risk nursing diagnosis
wellness diagnosis

DIAGNOSIS: STEP 2 OF THE NURSING PROCESS

Diagnosis is the second phase of the nursing process; it involves the classification of disease, condition, or human response based upon scientific evaluation of signs, symptoms, history, and diagnostic studies. Diagnosis is also referred to as _____, _____ _____ or _____ _____. These corresponding terms are used interchangeably.

During the assessment phase, nurses use critical-thinking skills and judgment to _____, _____, and _____ assessment data. _____, _____ _____, and strengths of the client are identified. In the diagnosis phase problems, potential problems, and strengths are _____ with an appropriate **nursing diagnosis**. Once labeled, the nursing diagnosis communicates specific health care needs about the client to other members of the health care team involved in care.

Nursing Tip

All activities preceding this phase are directed toward formulating the nursing diagnosis, that is, problem identification. All care planning activities following this phase are based on the nursing diagnosis, the identified problem(s).

Differentiating Between Medical and Nursing Diagnoses

A **medical diagnosis** is made by the _____ and refers to a disease, condition, or pathological state only a physician can treat. Examples of medical diagnoses are diabetes mellitus, congestive heart failure, hepatitis, cancer, and pneumonia. The medical diagnosis usually _____ _____ _____.

Nurses are _____ to follow the physician's order(s) and carry out pre-scribed treatments and therapies.

The term *nursing diagnosis* is used in three different contexts. First, it refers to the distinct _____ _____ in the nursing process, _____.
Next, nursing diagnosis applies to the _____. Nurses assign meaning to collected assessment data. Actual problems and problems the client is at risk for de-veloping are identified and appropriately labeled with a NANDA-approved nursing diagnosis. For example, a client is admitted into the hospital and medically treated for a heart attack (acute myocardial infarction). The physician prescribes treatment, such as diagnostic tests, therapies, and various medications. The nurse carries out the physician orders and monitors the client. During the assessment, the nurse may iden-tify that the client is experiencing anxiety over the medical diagnosis, fear and anxi-ety over an uncertain future, and difficulty sleeping. It is those problems which are labeled with nursing diagnoses: respectively, *Anxiety*, *Fear*, and *Sleep Pattern Distur-bance*. Nurses will intervene individually or collectively with the physician to resolve each response. Nurses understand the _____ needs of the client and use _____ _____, _____, and _____ _____ as physician-prescribed treatment and nursing interventions are carried out. Finally, a nursing diagnosis refers to one of many diagnoses in the _____ _____ established and approved by NANDA. A com-plete list of nursing diagnoses, NANDA taxonomy, can be found in Appendix A.

Characteristics of Nursing Diagnoses

Actual nursing diagnoses describe the client's _____ to a physical, sociocultural, psychological, and/or spiritual illness, disease, or condition.

For example, the physician diagnoses a client with a medical illness, pneumonia, and writes orders for hospital admission and treatment. During the initial interview and assessment, subjective and objective data are collected indicating the client is restless, hypoxic (reduced oxygen in inspired air), and too weak to cough productively. The nurse correctly identifies and labels one nursing diagnosis as *Impaired Gas Exchange*. Interventions will be planned and instituted by the nurse to improve the client's gas exchange at the cellular level, aiding in problem improvement or resolution.

Nursing diagnoses may communicate _____ _____ _____ resulting from a client's physical, sociocultural, psychological, and/or spiritual illness, disease, or condition, termed risk nursing diagnoses. For ex-ample, an elderly client experiencing vertigo and difficulty walking refuses to call for

TABLE 3:1 Determining Appropriate Interventions Using Critical Thought

> Mrs. Johnson, sixty-six years of age, is admitted after falling and fracturing her pelvis. Data are gathered through an interview and physical assessment. The client requests medication for pain. The pain she is experiencing is a physiological response to her injury. Using a NANDA nursing diagnosis, the response is labeled as *Acute Pain.*
>
> Mrs. Johnson's physician has written analgesic orders, as follows:
> - Demerol 50 milligrams, intramuscular, every four hours, as needed for severe pain
> - Vicodin one or two, by mouth, every four hours, as needed for moderate pain
> - Tylenol ES two, by mouth every four hours, as needed for mild pain
>
> *What decision-making questions should the nurse ask Johnson regarding her pain?*

assistance with ambulation. The appropriate potential problem would be identified and labeled as *Risk for Injury.*

Nursing diagnoses may _____ as the client's condition _____ or the problem _____ or becomes _____. Refer back to the example of the client diagnosed with *Impaired Gas Exchange.* Nurses carry out physician-prescribed treatment for pneumonia, e.g., administer antibiotics, provide hydration, etc., and the client's physical condition improves. One would expect gas exchange within the lungs to improve. In this case, the problem of *Impaired Gas Exchange* would probably be resolved.

Nursing diagnoses may _____ physician prescribed treatment, but are _____ and _____. For example, if the hospitalized client had undergone a surgical procedure, one would expect to find physician-ordered analgesics. Medication is one important method to treat pain. (See Table 3:1, which shows an example of an analgesic order that a physician would write.) There are also many _____ nonpharmacological nursing interventions which may be

Nursing Tip

A client's medical diagnosis remains the same for as long as the disease process is present, whereas nursing diagnoses often change as the client's responses change.

initiated to alleviate the client's pain, and which would complement physician-prescribed treatment. Examples include imagery, distraction, relaxation, and massage.

Actual nursing diagnoses are developed when an *existing response* to an illness, disease, or condition is present at the time of the nursing assessment. The problem actually _____. The client is demonstrating subjective and/or objective data to _____ the conclusion. Actual nursing diagnoses are based on the _____ of associated _____ and _____.

Example:
Hyperthermia, client's temperature is 104.6°F
Impaired Gas Exchange, client's oxygen saturation in arterial blood is ninety-two percent
Pain, client states pain level is "eight" on scale of one to ten
Anxiety, client states he is experiencing anxiety
Self-Care Deficit, client is unable to perform activities of daily living

Risk diagnoses are determined when a _____ problem may develop but has not yet occurred. NANDA defines risk diagnosis as "a clinical judgment made when a client is more vulnerable to develop the problem than others in the same or similar situations."

Example:
Any person admitted into the hospital is at risk for acquiring a nosocomial infection. However, a client medically diagnosed with cancer, who is receiving chemotherapy and whose immune system is depressed, will hold a higher risk than others will for developing a hospital-acquired infection. The nurse would appropriately label this potential problem as *Risk for Infection*. Once identified, the health care team can take deliberate action and initiate interventions to prevent the problem from occurring.

Example:
An active eighty-year-old female was admitted into the hospital two days ago after falling in her home and sustaining a pelvic fracture. Day one after surgical repair, the client is experiencing a great deal of pain and refuses to move. Immobility, advanced age, and the client's refusal to shift her weight place the client at a greater risk for developing pressure ulcers. The nurse appropriately labels this potential problem as *Risk for Impaired Skin Integrity* and plans interventions to prevent skin breakdown from occurring.

Nursing Tip

- *The same set of nursing diagnoses cannot be expected to occur with a particular disease or condition.*
- *A single nursing diagnosis may occur as a response to any number of diseases.*

Components of Actual Nursing Diagnoses

For *actual* nursing diagnoses, the problem statement consists of three components: _____, _____, and _____ _____. Each element has a specific purpose.

The problem is the identified label of a client's health problem or response to the medical condition or therapy for which nursing may intervene. The problem is also known as the _____ _____.

The etiology, written as _____ _____ (R/T) includes conditions most likely to be involved in the development of a problem. This factor becomes the _____ for nursing interventions. The etiology or _____ component of the nursing diagnosis identifies one or more probable causes of the abnormal response. The etiology gives _____ to the problem statement. In view of this fact, the nurse is able to individualize care. NANDA uses the term _____ _____ to describe the etiology or likely cause of the actual nursing diagnosis.

Defining characteristics, written _____ _____ _____ (AEB), are the clinical _____ and _____ which confirm the problem exists. This component reflects *how* the diagnosis or problematic response is _____.

Nursing Tip

Remember, for actual nursing diagnoses, there are subjective and/or objective data, evidence that the problem actually exists.

Example:
The following are examples of actual nursing diagnoses, including all components.

Scenario one: The nurse is caring for a client who was involved in a motor vehicle accident and sustained superficial skin trauma. The client's epidermal layer of skin on the right knee, forearm, and hand is excoriated, reddened, and bleeding as the result of sliding across a cement pavement.

_____

_____

_____

_____

_____

Scenario two: A family member brings a young man into the emergency department. He has been working outside in the extreme heat and humidity. He is unresponsive. His skin is red, hot, and dry. Assessment of the client's vital signs reveals: pulse 106, blood pressure 156/96, respiration 26 breaths/minute, and temperature 106°F.

_____

_____

_____

Scenario three: The client you are caring for has been medically diagnosed with a right cerebral vascular accident (stroke). He experiences partial paralysis on the left side of his body. He is unable to turn over while in bed without assistance and has demonstrated decreased muscle strength and control in the left extremities.

_____

_____

_____

_____

Nursing Tip

Differentiating among possible causes of an identified problem is essential. Each cause or etiology may require different nursing interventions (see Table 3:2).

Components of Risk Nursing Diagnoses

Risk nursing diagnoses are identified when the client is *at risk* for developing a problem. The problem statement consists of two components, the _____ and _____ _____. The term *risk factor* is used to describe the etiology of risk nursing diagnoses, because there are _____ subjective or objective data present. The actual problem *does not exist* at the time of assessment. However, due to clinical circumstances, the client is at risk for developing this specific problem or complication. Table 3:3 compares components of actual and risk nursing diagnoses.

Examples of Risk Nursing Diagnoses

- Cancer patient, *Risk for Infection*
  Risk Factors (R/T): inadequate secondary defenses, immunosuppression
- Client with surgical incision, *Risk for Infection*
  Risk Factors (R/T): inadequate primary defenses, invasive procedure

TABLE 3:2 Comparison of Same Nursing Diagnoses with Different Etiologies Requiring Different Interventions

Nursing Diagnosis	Client	Etiology	Nursing Interventions
Constipation	Jim Beason	Inactivity, insufficient fiber intake	• Encourage daily activity to stimulate bowel elimination • Teach components of high-fiber diet to improve bowel function
	Terry Fielder	Long-term laxative use	• Identify factors that may contribute to constipation, such as medications, reduced fluid intake, dietary habits • Instruct client on adverse effects of long-term laxative use
Ineffective Breast-feeding	Christi Lawrence	Inadequate sucking reflex in infant	• Assess infant's ability to latch on and suck effectively • Monitor maternal skill with latching infant onto the nipple
	Cheri Phillips	Inexperience, knowledge deficit	• Determine mother's desire and motivation to breast-feed • Evaluate mother's understanding of infant's feeding cues, such as rooting

- Client who is semiconscious, vomiting, *Risk for Aspiration*
  Risk Factors (R/T): reduced level of consciousness, vomiting
- Neonate unable to maintain his body temperature, parent does not keep the child covered, *Risk for Hypothermia*
  Risk Factors (R/T): extremes of age, inadequate clothing
- Unsteady gait, refuses to call for assistance, *Risk for Injury*
  Risk Factors (R/T): impaired mobility, lack of knowledge regarding safety precautions

TABLE 3:3 Comparison of Components in Actual and Risk Nursing Diagnoses

Actual Nursing Diagnosis	Risk Nursing Diagnosis
Three components: • Nursing diagnosis • Related factor(s) • Defining characteristics	Two components: • Risk nursing diagnosis • Risk factor(s)

Nursing Tip

For risk nursing diagnoses, there are no defining characteristics or as evidenced by, per se. Risk factors identify characteristics that make the client more vulnerable to developing a specific problem.

Wellness Nursing Diagnoses

NANDA defines wellness diagnosis as "a clinical judgment about an individual, family, or community in transition from a specific level of wellness to a higher level of wellness." Wellness nursing diagnoses require a one-part statement, for example, Potential for Enhanced Nutrition (client has expressed a desire for improved nutritional status).

Key Concepts

- Diagnosis is the second step in the nursing process.
- Nursing diagnoses are different than medical diagnoses, in that nursing diagnoses describe the *client's response* to a physical, sociocultural, psychological, or spiritual illness, disease, or condition.
- Nurses have legal and ethical responsibilities to both medical and nursing diagnoses.
- Nursing diagnoses may change as the client's health status changes.
- The two most common nursing diagnoses are *actual* and *risk for* nursing diagnoses.
- An actual nursing diagnosis includes three components: the problem (nursing diagnosis label), etiology (related to), and defining characteristics (as evidenced by).
- A risk nursing diagnosis includes two components: the potential problem (risk nursing diagnosis) and risk factors (related to).
- Wellness nursing diagnoses require a one-part statement. Wellness nursing diagnoses may be included in the care plan for individuals expressing desire for a higher level of wellness.

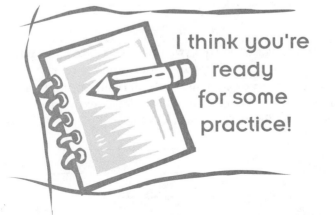

I think you're ready for some practice!

STUDENT PRACTICE: WRITING DIAGNOSIS STATEMENTS
Instructions

Read each case history and follow directions.

A. *Underline* abnormal subjective data and *circle* abnormal objective data.

B. Complete the *three-part* diagnostic statement that clearly describes the nursing diagnosis. In other words, what is the *related to* and *as evidenced by* information you will include with the nursing diagnosis?

1. Mr. Johnson is assessed and found to have the following signs and symptoms: awake, confused, and agitated. He responds to your questions, but sometimes he does not use appropriate terminology. He knows his name, but does not know he is in the hospital. He demonstrates a productive cough, which he spits in the emesis basin. The sputum is thick and yellow, with streaks of blood. Mr. Johnson states, "I smoked three packs of cigarettes a day for many years and I'm going to keep right on smoking!" Laboratory values reflect an elevated level of carbon dioxide in his blood. He is breathing twenty-four times per minute and using abdominal accessory muscles to breathe. He becomes short of breath (dyspnea) with minimal exertion. Capillary refill is sluggish, greater than three seconds. Both his hands and feet are pale and cold to touch.
(Nursing diagnosis, *Impaired Gas Exchange*)

_____

_____

_____

_____

2. John Burns demonstrates the following signs and symptoms: He states, "I have not felt like eating for about two months now." The nurse reviewed the previous week's admission record and found that the client's admission weight was 140 pounds. Today it is 134 pounds. The nurse reviews standards reflecting the recommended weight for the client's height and body frame. The client is fifteen pounds less than others his size. Mr. Burns states, "I can chew my food and swallow it, but I just don't have an appetite. I make myself eat at least one meal each day."
(Nursing diagnosis, *Altered Nutrition: Less Than Body Requirements*)

_____

_____

_____

_____

3. Mrs. Claire Jacobs was admitted two days ago to undergo surgery for a fractured hip. Her surgeon wrote the following orders: hips to remain adducted at all times, bed rest, physical therapy to assist with ambulation, and out of bed twice daily. She has limited passive range of motion in lower extremities.
(Nursing diagnosis, *Impaired Physical Mobility*)

_____

_____

_____

_____

4. Ms. Sharon Michaels, twenty-eight years of age, presents to the triage nurse at the local emergency department, complaining of severe generalized abdominal pain. She describes the pain as sharp and intermittent. She states, "Over the last four days, I haven't been able to have a bowel movement." She states that she is able to drink liquids and is urinating without difficulty. Bowel sounds are present in all four quadrants, however, they are hypoactive (decreased or quiet peristalsis). Abdomen is distended and firm to touch. She states, "Two weeks ago I fell and hurt my back. My doctor gave me a prescription for Tylenol #3 and I have been taking it every six hours for pain." She denies pain at the present time. Abdominal X rays reveal a large amount of stool in her lower colon. All other diagnostic tests are unremarkable.

(Nursing diagnosis, *Constipation*)

_____

_____

_____

_____

_____

_____

_____

STUDENT PRACTICE: IDENTIFYING CORRECTLY STATED NURSING DIAGNOSES

Instructions

For the nursing diagnoses listed below, identify those correctly stated. Use only NANDA nursing diagnoses.

1. _____ Risk for Constipation
2. _____ Risk for Hypothermia
3. _____ Risk for Pneumonia
4. _____ Need for Increased Fluids
5. _____ Ineffective Individual Coping
6. _____ Risk for Fluid Volume Deficit
7. _____ Altered Body Temperature
8. _____ Altered Self-Concept
9. _____ Anxiety
10. _____ Wound Infection
11. _____ Altered Communication
12. _____ Sudden Infant Death Syndrome
13. _____ Risk for Violence
14. _____ Altered Urinary Elimination
15. _____ Urinary Retention
16. _____ Pneumonia
17. _____ Airway Obstruction
18. _____ Cholecystitis
19. _____ Abdominal Pain
20. _____ Pain

21. _____ Anemia
22. _____ Ineffective Parenting
23. _____ Lung Cancer
24. _____ Risk for Injury
25. _____ Risk for Infection
26. _____ Confusion, Acute
27. _____ Ineffective Breast-Feeding
28. _____ Self-Care Deficit
29. _____ Incontinence, Bowel
30. _____ Congestive Heart Failure
31. _____ Cardiac Impairment
32. _____ Hopelessness
33. _____ Cardiac Output, Decreased
34. _____ Fear
35. _____ Stress, Acute
36. _____ Fluid Volume Excess
37. _____ Knowledge Impairment
38. _____ Crohn's Syndrome
39. _____ Noncompliance
40. _____ Confusion, Acute

STUDENT PRACTICE: PRACTICING STEP ONE AND STEP TWO OF THE NURSING PROCESS

Instructions

A. *Underline* abnormal signs and symptoms (do not underline complete sentences).
B. Above abnormal data, write O, if objective data and S, if subjective data.
C. Cluster data into related groups to identify and support each problem.
D. Label actual and risk problems using NANDA nursing diagnoses (include related to, as evidenced by, or risk factors, as appropriate).

General Information

Information Provided by: client
Name: Mrs. Janice Watson
Age: 46 years   **Sex:** female   **Race:** Caucasian
Admission Date/Time: March 15, 1999; 9:00 A.M.
Admitting Medical Diagnosis: Intractable Vomiting, Dehydration
Arrived on Unit by: wheelchair, from emergency department
Admitting Weight/Vital Signs: Temperature: 99.0°F; pulse: 76 bpm; respiration: 20 breaths/min; blood pressure: 112/78; weight: 145 pounds, height: five feet three inches
Client's Perception of Reason for Admission: client states she has had nausea and vomiting for four days.
Allergies: no known allergies (NKA)
Medications: no prescription medications; she took, "Pepto-Bismol, but I can't keep it down."

Assessment Data

Oxygenation: Reports no difficulty breathing; respirations 20 per minute. States she is a nonsmoker. Breath sounds are clear to auscultation bilaterally; no cough. Apical pulse 76, strong and regular; radial pulses are equal in strength and quality, however, easily obliterated. Pedal pulses are regular and equal in strength. Denies any chest pain. Brisk capillary refill of fingernail beds. No pedal, ankle, or leg edema noted.
Temperature: 99.0°F; denies having any fever over last few days
Nutritional/Fluid: She has an IV for hydration and electrolyte replacement in her right forearm. Five foot three inches, 145 pounds; weight has been relatively stable, until now. Reports weight loss of about five pounds since she became ill. States, "I haven't been able to eat for four days." Reports she normally eats two regular meals each day and has not been dieting. She complains of generalized abdominal cramping and is nauseated now. "I was trying to vomit in the emergency department, but there's just nothing in my stomach." Her skin turgor is inelastic, oral mucous membranes pink, but sticky.
GI/Elimination: Reports last bowel movement was two days ago; no diarrhea. Normal pattern is one bowel movement every day; states she urinated once yesterday. Abdomen is slightly distended and tender to palpation. Bowel sounds are present, but hypoactive.
Rest/Sleep: She states she has no difficulty sleeping at home, before she became ill. Denies use of sleeping aids or medications.
Pain Avoidance: Generalized abdominal cramping, described as sharp, intermittent, and rated as "six" on scale of one to ten. Nurse observes client holding her abdomen and stomach region.
Sexuality/Reproductive: Menstrual periods are usually regular, every twenty-eight

days. Client reports she had a tubal ligation after the birth of her second child about twenty years ago. Denies any concerns with sexual aspect of her life.

Activity: States she is active and has no problems. Client reports no aerobic activity, walks occasionally. Works as legal secretary for a well-known attorney. Enjoys going to the theatre with her husband and reading in her spare time.

Additional Data: The client is alert and oriented; responds appropriately to questions. Her eyes have a sunken appearance. Denies visual or auditory problems. The client's skin is intact, warm, and dry. Her hands tremble and she states, "Just leave me alone. I don't want to move."

Separate data into subjective and objective.

Subjective	Objective

Cluster data into groups of related data to determine problems.

_____

_____

_____

_____

_____

_____

_____

_____

_____

_____

Determine NANDA nursing diagnosis.

_____

_____

_____

_____

_____

_____

_____

Planning

"... in these and many other similar diseases the exact value of particular remedies and modes of treatment is by no means ascertained, while there is universal experience as to the extreme importance of careful nursing in determining the issue of the disease.

The most devoted friend or nurse cannot be there always. Nor is it desirable that she should.

It is as impossible in a book to teach a person in charge of sick how to manage, as it is to teach her how to nurse.

Conciseness and decision are, above all things, necessary with the sick. Let your thought expressed to them be concisely and decidedly mind must never be communicated to theirs, not even (I would rather say especially not) in little things.

What can't be cured must be endured, is the very worst and most dangerous maxim for a nurse which ever was made. Patience and resignation in her are but other words for carelessness or indifference—contemptible, if in regard to herself; culpable, if in regard to her sick."

Florence Nightingale

OBJECTIVES

Upon completion of this chapter, the student should be able to:

- Define the purposes of the planning phase.
- Identify and describe each component of the planning phase.
- Distinguish between goals and expected outcomes.
- Explain characteristics of nursing interventions and rationales.
- Discuss communication and documentation of the care plan.

KEY TERMS

care plan
client centered
dependent nursing
  intervention
discharge planning
expected outcome
goal

independent nursing
  intervention
interdependent
  nursing intervention
long-term goal
measurable
nursing intervention

planning
priority
rationale
short-term goal
strengths

PLANNING: STEP 3 OF THE NURSING PROCESS

Planning is the third phase of the nursing process. In prior steps, data were collected, analyzed, validated, and organized, and problems and strengths identified, then labeled with the appropriate nursing diagnosis. Nurses then develop a _____ of care, which establishes the proposed course of nursing action. The ultimate goal of the planning phase is to promote _____ or an _____ level of functioning for the client. Critical elements of planning include:

- _____
- _____
- _____
  _____
- _____
- _____

Scientific knowledge and understanding of the _____ needs of the client aid the professional nurse in effective planning. The purpose of this chapter is to explain the above critical components and to stress the importance of effective planning in promoting quality nursing care.

Planning begins as the nurse _____ the overall data collected during the assessment phase and the client's health care situation. Critical thought and problem solving are necessary skills when planning care. *Priority* problems requiring immediate attention are identified. *Strengths*, the client's *support system*, the health care *facility* itself, and available *resources* are considered, as well.

Priority problems are those appraised to be more important or life threatening. Priorities are dealt with before less critical problems. For example, Terrence Stewart was involved in an automobile accident and arrived at an emergency care center for treatment. Mr. Stewart began to experience symptoms suspiciously similar to an acute myocardial infarction (heart attack). In addition, he had sustained abrasions (skin scrapes) to his left arm and elbow during the accident. Obviously, the priority in this scenario is providing care to support the client's circulatory system (or cardiac function). The abrasions may be recognized as a problem, but they are less critical.

Strengths include physical, psychological, or personal characteristics. Strengths are thought to *promote* a higher or improved level of functioning. Examples of strengths include:

- physical strength: _____

_____

- psychological or personal strengths: _____

_____

- personal strengths: _____

_____

Facility refers to the health care delivery facility. The facility must be capable of providing the care necessary for a client. For example, if a client was a resident in a long-term care facility and sustained an injury requiring surgical intervention, this client will most likely require transfer to another facility equipped to provide surgical care. If another client began experiencing chest pain radiating to his left arm, and experienced nausea and shortness of breath (dyspnea), the most appropriate facility would be an acute care facility, not a health clinic.

Resources refer to the ways and means of obtaining health care. For example, is necessary equipment available at the facility? Does the client have transportation to obtain health care? Does the client have health insurance? Can the client afford to purchase medication or equipment prescribed?

Every aspect of the care plan should be *realistic* for both the client and the hospital, facility, or home care setting, depending on client needs. *What does the above statement mean?*

Purpose and Characteristics of Planning

Planning care must be individualized and realistic for each client. The purpose of planning includes promoting _____ in the client's present state of health or _____ the client's present health status. Planning facilitates _____ to diminished health, when an improved level of wellness is not possible, or promotes _____ and _____ to the client's deteriorating health. Steps involved in planning include:

_____

_____

_____

_____

_____

DETERMINING PRIORITIES

The first step in planning is determining **priorities** by recognizing problems that need immediate attention. Obviously, life-threatening situations must be given more urgency than non-life-threatening problems. Consider _____ _____ by encouraging input. Mutually setting priorities promotes compli-

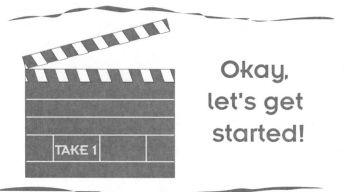

Okay, let's get started!

ance with care and the client's _____ _____ _____.
Table 4:1 shows common guidelines to assist in priority setting.

Consider *Maslow's hierarchy of needs*. Prioritize according to the basic physiological needs (oxygenation, nutrition, hydration, elimination, body temperature maintenance, and pain avoidance). Generally, _____ _____ _____ must be met sufficiently, before _____ _____ _____ (safe environment, security, love and belonging, and so on) are addressed.

Attention to more than one problem may occur simultaneously. For example, the

TABLE 4:1 Associating Maslow's Hierarchy of Needs with Priority Problems

Priority 1 Physiological needs	• Problems interfering with ability to maintain physiological life processes, such as ability to breathe, maintaining a patent airway, maintaining adequate circulation • Problems interfering with homeostatic physiological responses within the body, such as respiration, circulation, hydration, elimination, temperature regulation, nutrition • Problems interfering with ability to be free of offensive stimuli, such as pain, nausea, and other physical irritation
Priority 2 Safety/security	• Problems interfering with safety and security, such as anxiety, fear, environmental hazards, physical activity deficit, violence towards self or others
Priority 3 Love and belonging	• Problems interfering with love and belonging, such as sensory-perceptual losses, inability to maintain family and significant other relationships, isolation, loss of a loved one
Priority 4 Self-esteem	• Problems interfering with self-esteem, such as inability to perform normal daily activities of living, change in physiological structure or function of body or body part
Priority 5 Self-actualization	• Problems interfering with one's ability for self-actualization, such as positive personal assessment of life events, achieving personal goals

Now That We Have
Our "Priorities" In Order...
We Want to Look at
Establishing Goals

nurse may be performing interventions related to pain reduction and, at the same time, instructing and encouraging the client about proper use of an incentive spirometer, thus improving the client's oxygenation status.

Finally, priorities may include setting _____ and instituting _____ to prevent problems from occurring. Nurses often anticipate potentially serious problems that may arise without nursing intervention.

ESTABLISHING GOALS AND EXPECTED OUTCOMES

After priority problem identification, setting goals and expected outcomes follows. One overall goal is determined for each nursing diagnosis. Goals are:

- _____
- _____
- _____

Before we Get
Started on This
Journey...we Need
Direction!

Definition and Components of Goals and Expected Outcomes

The terms *goal*, *outcome*, and *expected outcome* are often used interchangeably. A goal is a general statement indicating the _____ or _____ _____ in the client's health status, function, or behavior. An expected outcome is more specific, describing the _____ through which the goal

TABLE 4:2 Application of Goals and Expected Outcomes

Nursing Diagnosis: *Body image disturbance*
Goal: Client will demonstrate acceptance of amputation and an ability to adjust to lifestyle change within six months.
Expected Outcomes:
• Looks at and touches area of missing body part
• Participates in wound/stump care
• Plans for prosthesis
• Returns to former social involvement
Nursing Diagnosis: *Impaired gas exchange*
Goal: Client will maintain a patent airway throughout hospitalization.
Expected Outcomes:
• Verbalizes understanding of oxygen administration and respiratory treatments
• Maintains adequate oxygenation and ventilation
• Remains free of signs of respiratory distress

will be _____. Refer to Table 4:2 for goal and expected outcome application examples.

Goals and expected outcomes must be measurable (able to be quantified). The client demonstrates a certain action within a specified time frame. The demonstrated _____ and _____ _____ are the yardsticks which allow the goal or expected outcome to be _____. As interventions, planned with goal resolution in mind, are carried out nurses determine how the client responds to each intervention. Favorable responses will most likely lead to attainment of goals and resolution of problems. Goals and expected outcomes provide the health care team with a clear understanding of what is to be accomplished. Goals and expected outcomes are client centered. The client (or part of the client) is expected to achieve a desired outcome.

Goals are constructed by focusing on problem _____, _____, and/or _____. A short-term goal is a statement identifying a _____ _____ _____ that can be achieved fairly quickly, usually within a few _____ or _____. A long-term goal indicates an objective to be achieved over a longer period, usually over _____ or _____. Long-term goals focus on overall greater expectations that may require ongoing health care attention. Discharge planning involves identifying long-term goals, thus promoting continued restorative care and problem resolution through home health, physical therapy, or various other referral sources (Figure 4:1).

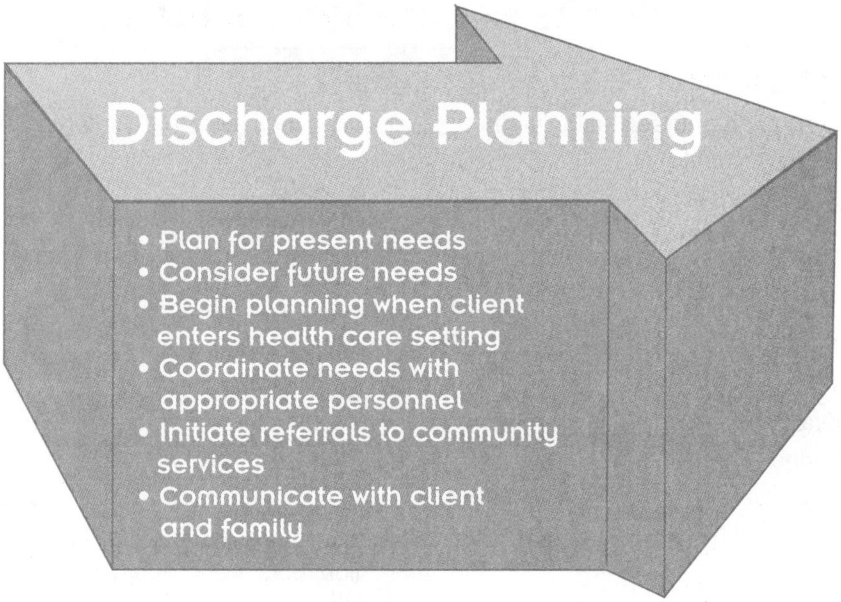

FIGURE 4:1 Goals for Discharge Planning

After the goal is stated, expected outcomes are identified. Expected outcomes are measurable steps indicating _____ toward _____ _____. For each nursing diagnosis and overall goal, there may be several expected outcomes. Both goals and expected outcomes include specific components when appropriately expressed (see Table 4:3 for examples of common mistakes in writing goals). Components include: _____.

- The subject identifies the person who will perform the desired behavior or meet the goal. Since goals are _____, _____, subject refers to the _____.

- Behavior describes *what* the client will do to achieve the goal (see Table 4:4) for examples of measurable verbs). Behavior can be _____, _____, _____, or _____. For example:
  - will verbalize
  - will ambulate
  - will report
  - will eat
  - will demonstrate

- The criteria of performance refer to the standards indicating the _____ of _____, such as how long, how far, how much. Criteria of performance may include a time limit, amount of activity, or description of the behavior to be followed.

Examples include:
  - understanding of medication regime
  - length of the hall
  - decrease in pain level of four or less

TABLE 4:3 Common Mistakes in Writing Goals

Incorrect	Correct
• Focus on the nurses action when writing the goal	• Goals must be client centered. The *subject* in the goal is the client, for example, *client will demonstrate correct self-administration technique of insulin injection within forty-eight hours of initial instruction.*
• Statement of unrealistic goal for client. For example, a client with advanced Alzheimer's, incontinent of urine, whose care plan goal reads: client will remain continent throughout hospitalization.	• Goals should be realistic. Ask yourself, can the client perform the stated action, thus achieving the goal within the stated time frame? For the incontinent client with advanced Alzheimer's, a more appropriate goal might be stated, client will maintain skin integrity as evidenced by use of continence aids to keep skin dry throughout shift.
• Goal lacks time frame	• The time frame indicates *when* the goal should be achieved. Otherwise, determination of the client's success or failure in achieving the desired result can not be evaluated. Appropriately stated goals require four components: subject (*the client*), behavior (*will maintain*), criteria of performance (*skin integrity*), and time frame (*throughout shift*). A fifth component, conditions, is optional. In the example above, *use of continence aids to keep skin dry,* is the condition.
• More than one task or behavior to be accomplished in one goal statement. For example, client will demonstrate a tolerable level of discomfort and will identify at least two alternative measures to reduce pain level within eight hours.	• Only one behavior should be specified for each goal. Goals will be more explicit and directly measurable.

- seventy-five percent of meal
- decreased blood pressure within forty-eight hours
- Conditions, *an optional component,* refer to the aid or conditions which facilitate the performance. Conditions may provide _____. They include experiences the client is expected to have before performing the behavior. For example:
  - with the assistance of physical therapy
  - with the administration of analgesics

TABLE 4:4 Measurable Verbs

Identify	Describe	Perform	Relate
State	List	Verbalize	Hold
Demonstrate	Share	Express	Sit
Exercise	Communicate	Stand	Discuss
Cough	Walk	Describe	Reestablish

- with assistance of family
- with use of medication and diet therapy

- The time frame refers to when the behavior should be accomplished, for example:

  - within forty-eight hours
  - by third postoperative day
  - within forty-five minutes
  - in twenty-four hours
  - within three weeks of medication therapy

WRITING GOAL AND OUTCOME STATEMENTS

The following are examples of goals stated correctly:

- Client will ambulate assisted by physical therapy to nurse's station and back to room twice daily.
- Client will verbalize understanding of medication regime prior to discharge.
- Client's skin will demonstrate no evidence of breakdown throughout hospitalization.
- Ms. James will lose two-and-a-half lbs. within three weeks by using prescribed American Heart Association Diet plan.
- Client will ambulate unassisted with crutches by discharge.
- Client will demonstrate correct injection technique by September 18.

STUDENT PRACTICE: WRITING GOALS
Instructions

For each nursing diagnosis write an appropriate goal. (Remember goal components.)

1. Joe Johnson has experienced intermittent nausea for approximately six months due to a possible gastric ulcer. He states, "I know I should eat, but when I eat, I hurt." He has lost twenty-eight pounds since his last annual checkup and weighs less than is ideal for his height. His nurse identifies the nursing diagnosis: *Altered Nutrition: Less than Body Requirements*; related to: inability to ingest nutrients as a result of biological factors; as evidenced by: reported food intake less than recommended daily allowance, weight loss of twenty-eight pounds over last year.

_____

_____

2. Hannah Miller, a neonate, is experiencing a fluctuation in her body temperature from normal to below normal range. Her nurse discovers that Hannah's mother does not keep her covered appropriately. The nurse identifies the nursing diagno-

sis: *Risk for Hypothermia*, risk factors: exposure to cool environment, inadequate clothing, extremes of age (newborn).

_____

_____

3. Mr. Cooper had abdominal surgery one day ago. He has a medical history of diabetes mellitus and must take morning and evening insulin subcutaneously. His nurse identifies the nursing diagnosis: *Risk for Infection*, risk factors: inadequate primary defenses (surgical incision/broken skin), increased environmental exposure, chronic disease, invasive procedures.

_____

_____

4. Mr. Sanders states he has been traveling out of the country. Since his return last week he has been experiencing abdominal cramping and several liquid stools. The nursing diagnosis identified is *Diarrhea,* related to: gastrointestinal disorder; as evidenced by: abdominal cramping, increased frequency of defecation, liquid stools.

_____

_____

5. Mrs. O'Conner was admitted to the hospital diagnosed with pneumonia. Assessment reveals bilateral wheezes in the midanterior lung fields and mild dyspnea. The nurse observes Mrs. O'Conner coughing up copious amounts of thick, yellow sputum. The nursing diagnosis is identified as *Ineffective Airway Clearance*, related to: tracheobronchial infection; as evidenced by: abnormal breath sounds (wheezes), productive cough, dyspnea.

_____

_____

Nursing Tip

Planning is
One . . . Identifying Priorities
Two . . . Setting Goals
And
Three . . . Planning Nursing Interventions

PLANNING NURSING INTERVENTIONS

After prioritizing problems and setting goals, nurses use problem-solving and decision-making skills in determining what _____ will aid in problem _____. Nursing interventions are specified _____ executed by the nursing team which benefit the client in a _____ _____.

> ## Nursing Tip
> *Interventions are actions carried out by nurses to meet goals and therefore, to resolve identified actual or potential problems.*

Interventions are _____ strategies to be implemented with problem _____ or _____ in mind.

Characteristics of Nursing Interventions

Nursing interventions are activities or actions planned by the nurse to produce problem resolution, problem reduction, or prevention of risk problems. Nursing interventions may be planned to assist the client accept his or her present state of health or illness. Nursing interventions specify activities to execute. They focus on the etiology of the problem and may determine _____ activities are to be carried out, _____ _____, and the _____ for each activity.

Nursing interventions are _____ to other nurses involved in the client's treatment by verbal or written report and through documentation of the plan, which promotes continuity of care.

Guidelines for Selecting Nursing Interventions

Appropriate interventions are selected using _____ provided by official nurse regulating organizations, such as individual nurse practice acts, state boards of nursing standards, and the Joint Commission on Accreditation of Healthcare Organizations' (JCAHO) standards for nursing care. Nurses must practice within the legal realm of nursing guidelines and boundaries. Furthermore, interventions must be _____ for the client and nurse, as well as for the facility. Nurses consider the client's _____ and _____ and the _____ and _____ of each intervention.

Classification of Nursing Interventions

Nursing interventions are classified according to three categories: _____ _____

Independent nursing interventions are nursing actions initiated by the nurse _____ _____ _____ or an order from another health care professional. They are actions _____ by state boards of nursing and nurse practice acts, which allow nurses to independently intervene depending on client needs. Interventions may ＿＿＿＿＿＿ activities of daily living, health education, health promotion, and counseling. For example, the environment may be managed by nurses to establish and maintain a safe, therapeutic environment, promote rest, reduce noise, maintain cleanliness, or manage environmental temperature.

Interdependent nursing interventions are actions developed in ＿＿＿＿＿＿ or ＿＿＿＿＿＿ with other health care professionals to gain another's viewpoint in determining an intervention most beneficial for the client. An example would be discussion of the client in an interdisciplinary conference for discharge planning, attended by the primary nurse or supervisor, home health care nurse, social worker, physical therapist, and dietician.

Nurses may consult with specialists when the problem cannot be resolved using their personal knowledge or skills. Specialists may be consulted to determine the best method for nursing diagnosis resolution, for example, consulting a dietician regarding a special diet.

Dependent nursing interventions are actions ＿＿＿＿＿＿ ＿＿＿＿＿＿ ＿＿＿＿＿＿ from a physician or another health care professional, such as a request for physician-prescribed medication orders. Likewise, nurses may question a previously written order based on knowledge of current client status or change in the client's condition, requesting clarification or new orders.

Nursing interventions are determined based on scientific principles and knowledge from behavioral and physical sciences. The nurse uses deliberate thought processes to determine actions which will aid in ＿＿＿＿＿＿, ＿＿＿＿＿＿, or ＿＿＿＿＿＿ of the cause or ＿＿＿＿＿＿ of the problem or nursing diagnosis. Therefore, interventions are developed from the ＿＿＿＿＿＿ of each nursing diagnosis.

Where Do Nursing Interventions Originate?

Depending on the client's problem, interventions may originate from the environment. Examples include:

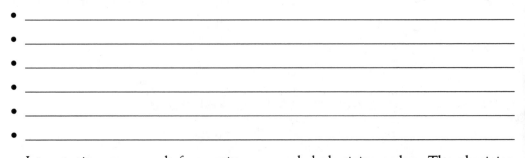

Interventions may result from written or verbal physician orders. The physician relies on the nurse's judgment and ability to carry out orders in a safe, effective manner. Nursing interventions may be written to complement the physician-prescribed treatments.

Nursing interventions may result from such client needs as health-related teaching, counseling, or referrals to other health care professionals. Interventions may involve specific nursing treatments or collection of ongoing assessment data related to client status. Other interventions may evolve from measures to take during basic care, such as suctioning, repositioning, assisting with nutrition, providing hygiene measures, assisting with activities of daily living, providing emotional support, or maintaining range of motion.

Example:
Nursing Diagnosis: *Activity intolerance*. R/T: bed rest, generalized weakness. AEB: verbalization of overwhelming lack of energy, dyspnea on exertion while performing activities of daily living.
Goal: *Client will verbalize improved level of energy when carrying out activities of daily living within one week.*

1. Assess ability to perform activities of daily living.
2. Evaluate adequacy of nutrition and sleep.
3. Schedule periods of uninterrupted time for client to rest throughout the day.
4. Assist client with activities of daily living as necessary. Promote and encourage ADL independence without causing exhaustion.

Interventions are prioritized according to the order in which they will be implemented or carried out. Several interventions should be identified for each goal.

Scientific Rationales

As previously explained, interventions are selected based on an understanding of scientific principles and psychosocial or developmental theories. Understanding of the human body and mind allows for certain _____ _____ when interventions are carried out. Rationales are the _____ _____ for which the intervention was chosen. When interventions are chosen, nursing students should identify and provide scientific rationale for each intervention. This action aids in further understanding of the theoretical and scientific knowledge of nursing.

Nursing Tip

Determine key words in interventions and diagnoses such as postsurgery and hypoxia. Rationales for these would be found in medical-surgical textbook chapters relating to any client undergoing surgery for any reason. Hypoxia is a postoperative complication for which the nurse must monitor.

Example:
You are caring for a client medically diagnosed with emphysema who refuses to quit smoking cigarettes.
Nursing diagnosis: *Noncompliance* (therapeutic regime)
Related to: client value system, health belief
As evidenced by: failure to adhere to health recommendations, evidence of exacerbation of symptoms
Goal: Client will communicate an understanding of disease process and treatment prior to discharge.
Nursing Intervention: Collaborate with client to implement a plan for smoking cessation.
Rationale: *Active participation in decision making about therapeutic regime may increase compliance.*

Scientific research has provided proof that a client who participates in health care decision making is more likely to be compliant. This data may be located in research articles, fundamental or foundation textbooks, nursing journals, and other resources. Identify the *key word,* such as decision making or compliance, and then locate the rationale in one of the resources or references.

Example:
For the client who had orthopedic surgery:
Nursing Intervention: Monitor airway and respiratory pattern every two hours for initial eight to twelve hours or until stable.
Rationale: *Most anesthetic agents depress respiratory rate and depth, thus interfering with oxygenation of the blood.*

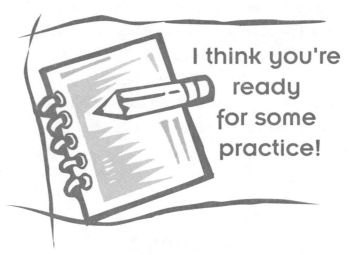

I think you're ready for some practice!

STUDENT PRACTICE: SCIENTIFIC RATIONALES
Instructions

Determine scientific rationales for each nursing intervention below.
Nursing Diagnosis: *Activity intolerance.* R/T: bed rest, generalized weakness; AEB: verbalization of overwhelming lack of energy, dyspnea on exertion while performing ADLs
Goal: *Client will verbalize improved level of energy when carrying out activities of daily living within one week.*

Nursing Interventions:

1. Assess ability to perform activities of daily living. _____

_____

_____

2. Determine cause of activity intolerance and determine if the cause is physical or motivational.

_____

_____

3. Encourage client to be out of bed. Increase activity gradually. _____

_____

_____

4. Allow clients sufficient time to carry out activities of daily living and give adequate rest periods between activities. Provide assistance as necessary:

_____

_____

COMMUNICATING AND DOCUMENTING THE CARE PLAN

The client's plan of care is documented according to hospital policy and becomes part of the client's permanent medical record. The care plan is shared with other members of the health care team who are actively caring for the client. The plan may be reviewed by the oncoming nurse or communicated in part during report.

KEY CONCEPTS

• Planning is the third phase in the nursing process. Critical elements of planning include identifying priority problems and interventions, setting realistic goals and expected outcomes, determining nursing interventions and rationales for each intervention, and finally, communication and documentation of the care plan.
• Establishing priorities may be guided by factors such as endangerment to life, client preferences, and Maslow's hierarchy of needs.
• The care plan is realistic and practical. It considers the client's values, beliefs, and strengths, as well as physical and psychological health.
• Planning individualized care for the client may promote improvement of health, preserve the client's present state of health, help the client to adjust to diminished or a decreasing level of health, or assist the client in accepting deteriorating health.
• A goal indicates the desired change in the client's health status. Goals are client centered and give direction to the care plan. Goals are constructed by focusing on problem prevention, resolution, or rehabilitation. Components of a goal statement include the subject, behavior, criteria of performance, conditions, and time frame.
• Expected outcomes are more specific than goals and describe the methods through which the goal is achieved.
• Goals and expected outcomes are used to measure the success of the care plan. Goals and expected outcomes are stated in a manner that makes them measurable.

- Nursing interventions are actions to be carried out by the nurse and are expected to benefit the client in a predictable manner. Interventions are developed to meet goal objectives and therefore aid in problem resolution.
- Nursing interventions are selected based on the nurse's understanding of scientific principles and psychological or developmental theories. Rationales are the underlying scientific reason for which the intervention was chosen.
- The nursing care plan is a formal written document that becomes part of the client's permanent medical record.
- Documentation and communication of the plan promotes continuity of care.

STUDENT PRACTICE: PLANNING AND OUTCOME IDENTIFICATION
Instructions

Using the scenario from chapter 3, Mrs. Janice Watson, medical diagnosis of Intractable Vomiting, Dehydration:

1. Complete all steps involved in planning and outcome identification. (See chart, Figure 4:2.)
2. Identify two or three priority problems. For each problem, determine one nursing diagnosis statement (label, related to, and as evidenced by), one goal, and three interventions with scientific rationale.

Name: _____ Date: _____

Care plan documentation form: For each nursing diagnosis, include related to, as evidenced by, or risk factors (if risk nursing diagnosis); one goal/expected outcome per nursing diagnosis; and at least three nursing interventions with scientific rationale for each. Evaluate goal/expected outcome when appropriate (one evaluative statement).

Nursing Diagnoses (R/T + AEB)	Goal	Nursing Interventions	Scientific Rationale	Evaluation
1.		1. 2. 3.	1. 2. 3.	
2.		1. 2. 3.	1. 2. 3.	

FIGURE 4:2 Care Plan Documentation Form

Implementation

"As the results of good nursing, as detailed in these notes, may be spoiled or utterly negatived by one defect, viz.: in petty management, or, in other words, by not knowing how to manage that what you do when you are there, shall be done when you are not there.

And she may give up her health, all her other duties, and yet, for want of a little management, be not one-half so efficient as another who is not one-half so devoted, but who has the art of multiplying herself.

To be "in charge" is certainly not only to carry out the proper measures yourself, but to see that every one else does so too; to see that no one either willfully or ignorantly thwarts or prevents such measures. It is neither to do everything yourself nor to appoint a number of people to each duty, but to ensure that each one does that duty to which he is appointed.

Always sit down when a sick person is talking business to you, show no signs of hurry, give complete attention and full consideration if your advice is wanted, and go away the moment the subject is ended.

Always sit within the patient's view, so that when you speak to him he has not painfully to turn his head round in order to look at you.

Be motionless as possible, and never gesticulate in speaking to the sick.

Never make a patient repeat a message or request, especially if it be some time after.

If a patient has to see, not only to his own but also to his nurse's punctuality, or perseverance, or readiness, or calmness, to any or all of these things, he is far better without that nurse than with her—however valuable and handy her services may otherwise be to him, and however incapable he may be of rendering them to himself."

Florence Nightingale

OBJECTIVES

Upon completion of this chapter, the student should be able to:

- Discuss the purpose of the implementation phase of the nursing process.

- Describe ways in which the care plan is implemented.
- Identify the relationship between assessment and implementation.
- Discuss communication and documentation of client response to interventions as they are implemented.
- Describe key components of recording and reporting, including data to document on the client's chart and data to report to oncoming personnel.
- Discuss confidentiality and the client's right to privacy.

KEY TERMS

confidentiality	implementation	PIE charting
documentation	Kardex	reporting
focus charting	narrative charting	

IMPLEMENTATION: STEP 4 OF THE NURSING PROCESS

Implementation is the fourth phase of the nursing process. During this phase, activities such as executing nursing interventions, performing an ongoing assessment of the client, and determining the client's response to executed interventions are observed, communicated, and documented. As with all prior steps of the nursing process, nurses demonstrate knowledge and understanding of physical and social sciences and apply analytical skills and deliberate thought processes to interpret client responses to interventions. Nurses participate in ongoing assessment as implementation takes place. This chapter discusses the purpose and characteristics of implementation, guidelines for reporting and recording, and the client's right to privacy and confidentiality.

Characteristics of Implementation

The implementation phase is directed at meeting the client's needs through _____ of interventions and _____ of client response. These actions ultimately result in health _____, _____ of _____, or _____ of _____. During implementation priority interventions for priority problems are executed first. When the client is encouraged to provide input in _____ _____ and priority _____, the client maintains a _____ of _____ and _____ is enhanced.

Nursing professionals monitor the client's response to treatment and therapies through means of _____ _____ and _____ with the client. Nurses _____ the client's response. Evaluation may include additional inquiry, such as reviewing laboratory results, progress notes, and collaborating with the physician and other nurses involved in the client's care. Accurate _____ and _____ of all pertinent data are necessary.

DOCUMENTATION

Several factors are considered for documentation to be effective. Documentation is the process of preparing a record reflecting the assessment data and both the client's health status and response to care. Depending on the facility, various formats may be used. Appendix B includes sample documentation forms. Guidelines for documentation include:

- Document on the appropriate record.
- Verify name before entries are documented.
- Each page should include identification.
- Use common vocabulary and approved abbreviations or symbols.
- Write legibly.
- Write only in permanent ink.
- Date and time each entry.
- Sign each entry with your name and credentials.
- If an error is made, draw one single line through the entry, initial, and write *incorrect entry* over the error and line.
- Never erase or use correction fluid on entry corrections.
- Document thoroughly in sequential order.
- Document at appropriate intervals throughout the shift.
- Identify documentation entries that are out of time-sequential order. Label as *late entry* by the entry time.
- Document the facts: what you observe, hear, feel, smell, or can measure. Do not make assumptions or state opinions.
- Document telephone calls made or received concerning the client's care.
- When using a checklist format, fill in all areas on the form completely. When unable to provide an accurate description, refer the reader to the narrative note entry.
- Never change another person's entry.
- Never leave a space between entries or leave a partial space midline. Draw one single line from the end of your entry to the end of the line and initial.
- Document within your facility's documentation guidelines.

Figure 5:1 compares examples of correctly and incorrectly documented data on a twenty-four-hour record.

Documentation Methods

Depending on your facility, many different systems may be utilized for documentation purposes: narrative, PIE, focus, and others. Always be familiar with your facility's documentation policies and procedures and document within those guidelines.

Narrative Charting

Narrative charting refers to a traditional documentation system. The nurse records _____ _____ relating to the client as progress notes, some-

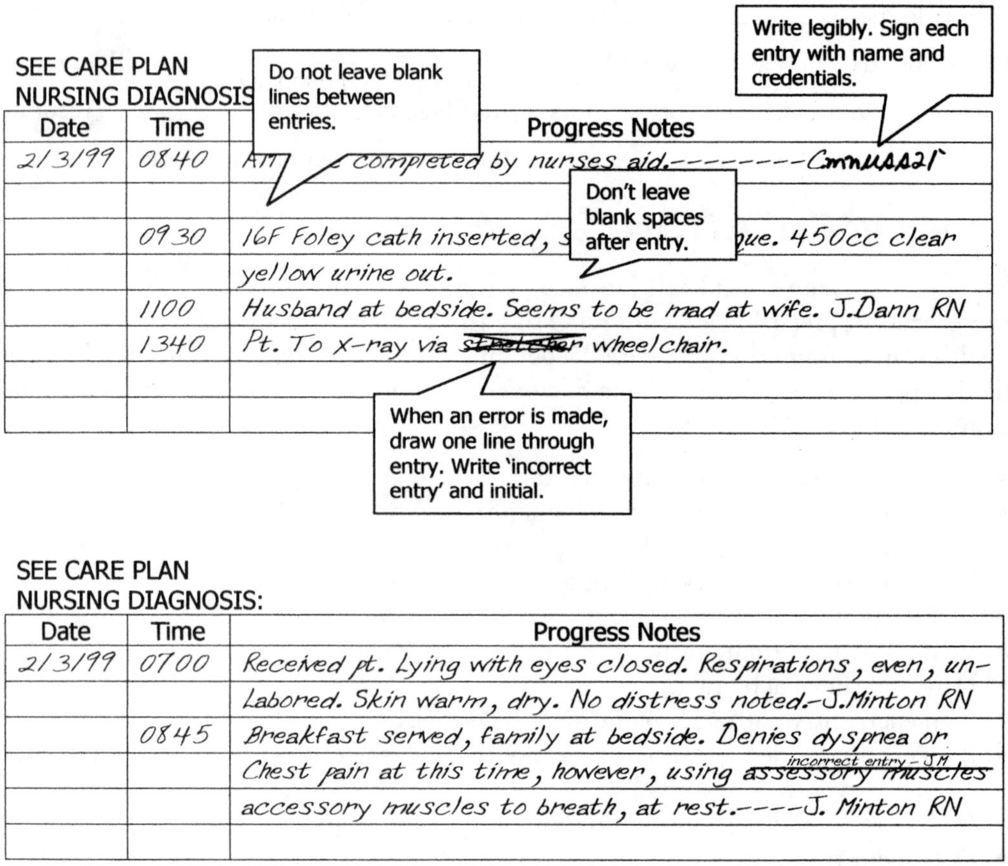

FIGURE 5:1 Examples of Incorrect and Correct Documentation.

times supplementing with flow sheets. Narrative documentation is a sequential description, which includes: _____

_____

_____

Be specific and descriptive when documenting narrative notes. See the acronym CHARTING in Table 5:1 for data to include.

PIE Charting

PIE (problem-intervention-evaluation), **charting** organizes information according to _____ the client is experiencing, _____ performed, and _____ of client response. Assessment flow sheets and progress notes are maintained on a daily basis. Initial assessment determines problems, labels them as nursing diagnoses, and numbers them for future reference. For example, when the nurse documents data regarding problem one, the entry notation begins with *P #1*. For interventions performed in relation to problem one, the entry notation begins with *I-P #1*, followed by the entry. When the nurse evaluates the response to an intervention for problem one, the entry notation begins with *E-P #1*, followed by the evaluation entry, and so on. Figure 5:2 shows an example of PIE documentation.

TABLE 5:1 Documentation to Include While Charting

Condition: current condition of the client, physically, emotionally; condition of wounds/dressings; change in condition of client

Happenings: abnormal or variations from usual routine; visits from family, physician, discharge instructions

Additions: changes to the care plan; abnormal laboratory values

Response: to interventions carried out, reactions or response to medications administered, reports received or given to other personnel

Treatments, transfers, transport to other departments

Invasive procedures performed

Notes: refers to narrative notes when the flow sheet is not enough

Good job!

FOCUS Charting

The **focus charting** system involves documentation of three categories: *data, action,* and *response*, or DAR. Figure 5:3 shows an example of a focus charting system. The *D* or *data* category is the _____ of the entry. Each focus may include specific identified problems stated as nursing diagnoses or may identify the topic of the entry.

Examples of data may include:

- a nursing diagnosis _____

- subjective or objective data _____

SEE CARE PLAN
NURSING DIAGNOSIS:

DATE	TIME	NOTES
12/15/99	1330	P#1 = Complaints of acute pain to right lower quadrant
		abdomen. Rates as "7" on scale of 1 to 10.
		IP#1 = adm. Analgesics as prescribed. Monitor quality,
		location, intensity, & frequency. Document. Encourage
		diversional activities, such as, music, focus breathing
		reading, etc. Advise to request analgesic prior to pain
		Becoming intense------------------------W.Seaback RN
		EP#1 = pain resolves. Client requests analgesics when
		pain level "4" or less on scale of 1 to 10. Participates
		in diversional activities. VS remain within normal limits.
		Client reports further symptoms._____ W.Seaback RN
12/13/99	1330	P#2 = Risk for Infection RT surgical incision
		IP#2 = sterile wound care qd, as per MD orders.
		Monitor wound for signs of redness, edema, drainage,
		odor, approximation. Monitor for temp elevation. Adm.
		Antibiotics as ordered.----------------W.Seaback RN
		EP#2 = incision heals without evidence of infection. No
		temp elevation.------------------------W.Seaback RN

FIGURE 5:2 PIE Charting Example.

SEE CARE PLAN
NURSING DIAGNOSIS:

Date	Time	Focus	Progress Notes
5/3/99	0945	Consti-pation	D: Pt states no BM for 4 days. Abdominal cramping. Bowel sounds hypoactive X 4 quads
	1015		A: administered 1000 cc warm, tap-water enema. Advised to hold as long as possible.
	1055		A: assisted to bedside commode. Call bell within reach.---------------W.Seaback RN
	1100		R: Client expelled large amount of dark, brown, formed stool, large amount of liquid and flatus.---------------W.Seaback RN
	1130		A: assisted into bed. Provided perineal care. D: excoriation noted to perineal area. Skin barrier applied. -------------W.Seaback RN
	1300	Nutri-tion	D: client ate 75% of soft mechanical diet. No nausea at this time.------W.Seaback RN

FIGURE 5:3 FOCUS Charting Example.

- client behavior _____
- change in the client's condition _____
- a significant event _____
- a special need _____

The A or *action* category includes nursing actions based on _____ of the client's _____. An example is administering an analgesic in response to the client's subjective statement of severe pain. The action entry includes the executed intervention. Actions may also include changes to the care plan deemed necessary, resulting from the nurse's assessment.

The *response* category (R) describes the client's response to nursing care, medical care, or specific interventions. In the example of administering an analgesic for severe pain, the response entry might include a statement noting severe pain was resolved.

Kardex

A **Kardex** is a condensed reference tool which includes _____ client care information. The Kardex is often used during _____ reports providing cues regarding pertinent information to discuss or relay. The Kardex may also be utilized as a _____ _____ throughout the shift.

When a client is admitted onto the nursing unit, data from the physician's admitting orders are generally penciled onto the card. As new physician orders are received, the Kardex is updated to reflect the change. A sample Kardex is shown in Appendix B.

Information contained on the Kardex may vary in different facilities; however, the Kardex often includes data such as:

- client data: name, age, sex, height, weight
- emergency data: name of contact person, relationship, address, telephone number
- daily diagnostic examinations, scheduled examinations or surgery
- medical diagnoses: admitting and history
- nursing diagnoses: by priority
- medical orders: diet, DNR (do not resuscitate) status, isolation, restraints, invasive procedures, vital sign parameters, activity, treatments, such as sitz bath or anti-embolytic stockings
- special therapies: respiratory therapy, physical therapy, occupational therapy
- routine medications including dosage amounts, times, intravenous solutions and medication, and as-needed medications

REPORTING

Reporting includes _____ _____ of facts regarding the client's health status and ongoing care provided. Thought should be given to what data are necessary to report. Data are _____, _____, and _____ to the appropriate person. Table 5:2 identifies an acronym, RECEIVE, with examples of data to include while reporting. Verbal reports may be required in a variety of situations, such as reporting to:

- oncoming shift personnel
- the receiving unit personnel if the client is transferred

TABLE 5:2 Information to Include in a Verbal Report

Reporting: facts, not opinions. Report objectively, accurately, be concise and complete.

Essential information about the client, such as name, age, sex, admission medical diagnosis, and pertinent history data.

Condition: current condition, such as diet, nothing by mouth (NPO), do not resuscitate (DNR) status, response to administered medication, Foley catheter, IV solution and site, orientation, prescribed activity level, fluid restriction, assistance needed by client, current teaching and client response, etc.

Extra medications, such as last prn (as needed) pain medication administered, preoperative medications on call or administered, medications to be given dependent on laboratory values. For example, "Give 20 mEq KCl for potassium <3.0."

Identify priorities relating to care, upcoming procedures, recurring laboratory tests, diagnostic tests completed, and results if known. Identify activities completed and those to be completed.

Values: such as last blood glucose level, vital sign parameters, abnormal vital signs, intake and output amounts, etc.

Exceptional report given!

- personnel in another facility when the client is discharged from one facility to be admitted to another

CONFIDENTIALITY

Information obtained from or about the client is considered to be *privileged* and, in most cases, cannot be disclosed to a third party. Clients have a legal and ethical _____ _____ _____. As a student or practicing nurse, you have a legal and ethical responsibility for protecting client _____. State laws ensure no one will reveal the client's confidential information without permission. Nurses should not disclose information about the client's status to other clients or staff not involved in the client's care. Nurses should not discuss any client's condition in inappropriate settings, such as the cafeteria or elevator.

> **Nursing Tip**
>
> *Always maintain client* **confidentiality.** *What does this term mean to you?*

KEY CONCEPTS

- Implementation is the fourth step in the nursing process. During implementation, nursing interventions are executed and the client's response is observed, communicated, and documented.
- As nurses interact with the client, assessment continues throughout each phase of the nursing process. New data are collected as the client responds to treatment, therapies, and nursing interventions.
- Client response's are reported to other health care professionals involved in the client's care and recorded in the twenty-four-hour client care record (nurse's notes).
- Nurses are ethically and legally obligated to protect client confidentiality.

STUDENT PRACTICE: DOCUMENTATION
Instructions

Read the brief vignette below.

A. Rewrite data in *narrative* documentation format.
B. Rewrite data in *focus* documentation format.

Complete sentences are not necessary.

Vignette: This morning when day shift began Mr. James was lying in bed with his eyes closed. When the nurse touched his arm, his skin was warm and dry. Mr. James's respirations were even and unlabored. He did not appear to be in any distress. Report was completed at 0715. When breakfast was served, around 0815, he was watching television. Mr. James complained of muscle spasms to his right lower calf [client recently fractured right tibia]. Capillary refill to his right great toe is less than two seconds. Feet are warm to touch and he moves them without difficulty. Skin condition around the cast edges is intact and without evidence of skin breakdown. Dr. Martin was called on the telephone at 0830 to advise of muscle spasms and to request new orders. Dr. Martin was in to see the client at 0955. He wrote an order for Mr. James to receive a new medication to reduce muscle spasms. Discharge orders were written. Mr. James states his wife will arrive within the hour for completion of discharge.

A: Narrative Documentation:

Date	Time		

B: Focus Documentation:

Date	Time	Focus	

STUDENT PRACTICE:
CHANGE-OF-SHIFT REPORT
Instructions

Locate Student Practice case scenario for client Mrs. Janice Watson in chapter 3. Using the data provided, determine information that would be necessary to report during change of shift.

_____

_____

_____

_____

_____

_____

_____

_____

_____

_____

_____

_____

_____

_____

NOTES

Evaluation

"A careful nurse will keep constant watch over her sick, especially weak, protracted, and collapsed cases, to guard against the effects of the loss of vital heat by the patient himself.

Now the medical man who sees the patient only once a day or even only once or twice a week, cannot possibly tell this without the assistance of the patient himself, or of those who are in constant observation on the patient. The utmost the medical man can tell is whether the patient is weaker or stronger at this visit than he was at the last visit. I should therefore say that incomparably the most important office of the nurse, after she has taken care of the patient's air, is to take care to observe the effect of his food, and report it to the medical attendant.

It is quite incalculable the good that would certainly come from such sound and close observation in this almost neglected branch of nursing, or the help it would give to the medical man.

Questions, too, as asked now (but too generally) of or about patients, would obtain no information at all about them, even if the person asked or had ever information to give. The question is generally a leading question; and it is singular that people never think what must be the answer to this question before they ask it . . . leading question always collect inaccurate information.

And nothing but observation and experience will teach us the ways to maintain or to bring back the state of health. It is often thought that medicine is the curative process. It is no such thing; medicine is the surgery of functions, as surgery proper is that of limbs and organs. Neither can do anything but remove obstructions . . . surgery removes the bullet out of the limb which is an obstruction to cure, but nature heals the wound . . . medicine, so far as we know, assists nature to remove the obstruction, but does nothing more. And what nursing has to do in either case, is to put the patient in the best condition for nature to act upon him."

Florence Nightingale

OBJECTIVES

Upon completion of this chapter, the student should be able to:

• Discuss the purpose of evaluation related to the nursing process.

- Identify characteristics of the evaluation phase and how to document evaluation.
- Discuss the relationship between assessment and evaluation.
- Identify how to evaluate effective goal achievement.
- Discuss when it is necessary to modify, revise, or discontinue portions of the care plan.

KEY TERMS

discontinue	goal attainment	revision
evaluation	modification	
evaluative statement	observation	

EVALUATION: STEP 5 OF THE NURSING PROCESS

Evaluation is the fifth phase of the nursing process. This step takes a critical look at the *results* of implemented nursing interventions. Although evaluation is the final step described in the nursing process, it is interwoven throughout all other steps. Evaluation involves critical analysis of the plan, beginning with initial data collection and continuing through implementation. Like assessment, evaluation is continuous and ongoing. Interventions and client responses are evaluated with questions. For example: Is the client progressing toward goal resolution? Have goals been met? Is this portion of the plan complete and no longer a problem for the client? Have goals been partially met or not met? When the client is not progressing as expected, answers are sought to determine why.

This chapter describes the purpose, characteristics, components, and methods for evaluation. The chapter also discusses evaluation of goal achievement, as well as determination of how and when to revise, modify, or discontinue the care plan.

Evaluation Purpose

The purpose of the evaluation phase is to estimate the _____ of _____ _____ and the _____ of _____ provided. Nurses evaluate client _____ to determine _____ the care plan is working or _____ _____ the care plan is working, and whether the client is progressing toward _____ _____ and _____ _____.

Characteristics of Evaluation

The evaluation phase and the assessment phase are similar in that they are both _____ and _____. When the client enters the health care continuum, initial assessment data are collected to establish a _____. Assessment, reassessment, and evaluation continue as *long as care is provided*. Client response is compared to _____ stated in the _____ _____, for example, reversal of symptoms, improved energy level, proper use of equipment, or reduced pain. Evaluation focuses on the _____ between the care provided and the client's progress toward _____ achievement.

In addition, the care plan is evaluated for its appropriateness and effectiveness. The nurse _____ the success of the previous steps of the nursing process and examines the client's response to interventions and medical treatment or therapies. Evaluation aids in _____ of the quality of nursing care provided at an institution or agency and helps determine if _____ to other resources, _____, or _____ may be necessary. Positive and negative factors are identified which affect the client's response. Questions asked may include:

- Were the expected outcomes achieved?
- Is the plan appropriate?
- Should the plan be modified or terminated?

The evaluation phase serves as a self-check to determine if the documented plan is working and if more might be accomplished. _____ results indicate the plan is working and is effective in meeting the client's goals. _____ results indicate goals are not met or only partially met; therefore, the identified etiology—hence, problem—is not being resolved. When documented, evaluation is stated in _____ or _____ _____. Refer to Figure 6:1 for an example of how evaluation is documented in a care plan.

Nursing Diagnosis	Goal Statement	Nursing Interventions	Scientific Rationale	Evaluation
Parenting, Altered R/T: lack of knowledge about child development AEB: Statements of inability to meet child's needs, role inadequacy, frustration	Client will report comfort with role expectations within one week.	1. Assist with identifying deficits/ alterations in parenting skills	1. Counseling involves a mutual exchange of ideas and provides a basis for problem solving.	Client reports that he is more comfortable in role expectations.

FIGURE 6:1 Documenting Evaluation of the Care Plan.

EVALUATION OF GOAL ATTAINMENT

The purpose of developing a care plan and providing nursing care is to assist the client in problem _____, _____, or _____ of one's present state of health. Goals and expected outcomes are written focusing on the etiology or cause of the problem. Once the cause is removed or resolved, the problem should be eliminated or at least should become more manageable. Therefore, evaluation of goal attainment will determine whether the _____ of the care plan was accomplished. The client's behavior or physiological _____ is compared to the behavior or response specified in the _____. Effective communication and observation are skills applied by the nurse. The client is observed for subtle or acute changes in physiological condition, emotional status, or behavior. Observation occurs through one's senses: _____, _____, _____, and _____. As actions are carried out and tasks are completed, the client's response is _____ and _____ as new data are obtained.

> ### Nursing Tip
>
> *Degrees of goal attainment include: the goal is met, partially met, or not met.*

Review of Goals and Expected Outcomes

A **goal** is the overall desired _____ in the client's health _____ or _____. Goals are stated in general terms. **Expected outcomes** are stated in more _____ terms. Both are directed toward the same destination. Expected outcomes may be thought of as more manageable targets advancing the client toward goal attainment. Goals and expected outcomes express _____ to be accomplished within a specified _____ _____. Once the behavior is demonstrated, advancement toward problem resolution is indicated. As hospital stays become shorter, many clients are discharged before all goals are met.

Care Plan Revision, Modification, or Discontinuation

As the client responds to treatment, therapies, and nursing interventions a change in the care plan may be warranted. Critical thought questions are asked:

- Has the expected outcome occurred?
- Is the client progressing as expected?
- Has there been a change in the client's condition?
- Is the client's health status improving?

REVISION or MODIFICATION

Progress toward goal attainment most likely indicates that appropriate interventions were planned and instituted. In this case, the client will continue to be monitored. Revisions (rewriting or amending) or modifications (alterations from the original) to the care plan are expected, however, as the client _____ to a _____ level of wellness. The care plan is revised or updated to reflect the client's changing needs.

Lack of progress toward goal attainment may indicate the care plan needs revision or modification as well. Unmet and partially met goals _____ the nursing process sequence. _____ of the client should begin. Once again, the nurse uses critical thought and judgment as collected data are _____, _____, and _____. Problems are _____ and _____ as nursing diagnoses. _____ is determined, and so on. All planning is _____ to that previously determined. **Modifications** to the care plan care are made where needed. Using analytical skills, the nurse examines each phase of the nursing process sequence:

* Was assessment thorough and data organized, verified, and interpreted?
* Were nursing diagnoses developed and prioritized appropriately?
* Are goals specific, measurable, and realistic?
* Were nursing interventions appropriate and prioritized? Did they address the goal to be accomplished?
* Did the client and family participate in goal setting and evaluation?
* Have assessment and evaluation been ongoing?
* Were revisions of the care plan documented as the needs of the client changed?
* Has effective communication regarding the care plan taken place from nurse to nurse?
* Does documentation reflect interventions, response, and the client's status?

DISCONTINUATION

Finally, when goals or desired outcomes are determined as *having been achieved* and the client no longer requires nursing assistance in this area, the nurse discontinues that portion of the care plan. Nurses continue to reassess the client for possible return of symptoms. For example, if the nursing diagnosis *Constipation* were resolved and no longer a valid concern to the client, the nurse would continue to assess function of the gastrointestinal tract.

Ideally, when preparing the client for discharge, it is appropriate to evaluate the status of each nursing diagnosis prior to discharge. An evaluative statement is written, identifying the client's partial progress toward goal _____ and problem _____. The care plan is revised for home and follow-up care. This plan is _____ in discharge instructions and _____.

NOTES

KEY CONCEPTS

- Evaluation is the fifth step of the nursing process. Although it is the final step, evaluation is interwoven throughout the entire nursing process sequence. Evaluation is continuous and cyclic in nature.
- The purpose of evaluation is to judge the effectiveness of chosen interventions, nursing care, and the quality of care provided.
- As evaluation takes place, assessment of the client continues. Evaluation of goal attainment compares the client's behavior or response to the behavior or response specified in the stated goal. It is this behavior and stated time frame that make goals measurable.
- Degrees of goal attainment include: the goal was met, partially met, or not met.
- As the client progresses toward a higher level of wellness, revisions or modifications to the care plan are expected. When specific problems have been resolved and no longer require intervention from the nurse, this portion of the care plan may be discontinued. Evaluation in the previously problematic area continues for possible return of signs or symptoms.

STUDENT PRACTICE: EVALUATION
Instructions

Answer the following questions.

1. What three essential cognitive skills are practiced in all steps of the nursing process? Define each skill.

    A. _____

    _____

    _____

    B. _____

    _____

    _____

    _____

    C. _____

    _____

    _____

    _____

2. Give one example of how the nurse may employ critical thinking in the following vignette: As the nurse entered the client's room, the client was holding her mid-chest or sternum area. The client was breathing faster than usual.

    _____

    _____

    _____

    _____

    _____

    _____

_____

_____

_____

3. What is the difference between assessment and evaluation?

_____

_____

_____

_____

_____

_____

_____

_____

_____

4. What are the similarities between assessment and evaluation?

_____

_____

_____

_____

_____

_____

_____

_____

_____

5. How is evaluation documented on the care plan?

_____

_____

_____

_____

_____

_____

_____

_____

_____

6. What is the purpose of evaluation?

_____

_____

_____

_____

_____

_____

_____

7. What does goal attainment mean in relation to evaluation and the nursing process?

_____

_____

_____

_____

_____

_____

_____

_____

8. When is the care plan or portions of the care plan revised, modified, or discontinued?

_____

_____

_____

_____

_____

_____

_____

_____

_____

_____

_____

Putting It All Together!

"If I have succeeded in any measure in dispelling this illusion, and in showing what true nursing is, and what it is not, my object will have been answered.

The everyday management of a large ward, let alone of a hospital, the knowing what are the laws of life and death for men, and what the laws of health for wards—are not these matters of sufficient importance and difficulty to require learning by experience and careful inquiry, just as much as any other art?

It is true we make "no vows." But is a "vow" necessary to convince us that the true spirit for learning any art, most especially an art of charity, aright, is not a disgust to everything or something else? Do we really place the love of our kind (and of nursing, as one branch of it,) so low as this one?"

Florence Nightingale

OBJECTIVES

Upon completion of this chapter, the student should be able to:

- Apply the steps of the nursing process to the provided scenario.
- Discuss each step of the nursing process, actions taken by nurses during each step, and the rationale of each action as it is applied.
- Identify how critical thinking is an important element of the nursing process.

APPLICATION OF THE NURSING PROCESS

The nursing process is a cyclic, ongoing method of providing client-centered care. It is a tool used by nurses to promote organization and utilization of the steps to achieve desired outcomes, that is, goal attainment and problem resolution.

As the client enters the health care system, nurses are involved in decision making. Care is planned for the client based on data continuously collected and analyzed. Initial data collected become the database used for comparison of future data.

Nurses use skills vital to all steps of the nursing process: critical thinking, problem solving, and decision making. Critical thinking is a purposeful thought process, in which deliberate questions are asked in search of meaning of data. Nurses solve problems by analyzing collected data in order to understand and make decisions regarding client needs. Decisions are made based on the nurse's understanding of scientifically based theories and knowledge of standards. These skills and others are employed as nurses interact with clients. Each interaction is an opportunity for the nurse to assess and evaluate client responses to care and medical treatment, as well as the effectiveness of care.

This chapter presents a review discussion of the nursing process. The nursing process steps are applied to a sample scenario, as if providing care to a client. A final care plan appears at the end of the chapter (Figure 7:1).

STEP 1: ASSESSMENT

Assessment includes _____, _____, _____, _____, _____, and _____ of data. Initial data gathered during an _____, physical _____, and _____ of diagnostic studies become the client database. This data may be used for _____ as additional data are collected. Once the client enters the health care system, other sources of data may include nursing records, medical records, verbal and written consultations, relevant literature regarding the client's illness, standards indicating normal functioning against which the client is compared, and other members of the health care team working with the client. _____ is a continuous process of collecting data to identify health problems or strengths of the client and perpetuates as long as there is a need for _____ _____.

Two categories of data are collected, subjective and objective. *Subjective* data include _____ made by the client, such as _____, _____, or _____. *Objective* data include signs which are _____, _____, or _____ by someone other than the person experiencing them. Each category _____ and _____ the other.

Collected assessment data are recorded using various tools designed for that purpose. Tools should consider all aspects of the client including _____, _____, _____, _____, and _____ well-being. Any tool format is acceptable, as long as it is thorough and comprehensive and considers the client's _____ age.

As data are collected, verified, and validated for accuracy, the nurse assigns meaning and groups data into clusters. _____ _____ is used to determine the _____ of facts, to find _____, and to determine if further data are needed. Related subjective and objective data are _____ together supporting the fact that a health problem exists that requires intervention.

Client Scenario

General Information

Information Provided by: client
Name: Tom Norman
Age: sixty-seven years   **Sex:** male   **Race:** African American
Admission Date/Time: November 22, 1999 / 15:45
Admitting Medical Diagnosis: rule out cerebral vascular accident (R/O CVA)
Arrived on Unit by: wheelchair from emergency department
Admitting Weight/Height/Vital Signs: weight 165 pounds, height five feet ten inches; blood pressure 152/84; pulse eighty-eight; temperature 99.2°F; respiration twenty
Client's Perception of Reason for Admission: severe headaches, weakness to left arm and left leg. Client states, "I have had this headache for three days. This morning, when I woke up, I realized I couldn't move my arm or leg. I think it has gotten better, but I don't know. My doctor told me to go to the emergency department. Can you give me something for this headache?" The nurse observes that the right corner of the client's mouth droops slightly and he has some difficulty pronouncing some words.
Allergies: aspirin (ASA), iodine
Medications: no prescription medications; he takes Tylenol for headaches and occasionally something for indigestion

Assessment Data

Oxygenation: Reports mild difficulty breathing when he arrived at the emergency department; oxygen is being administered via nasal cannula at two liters per minute; states he is a nonsmoker; breath sounds clear to auscultation bilaterally; no cough present; apical pulse eighty-eight, regular; radial pulses equal, regular, strong; left pedal pulse with decreased strength, regular rate and rhythm; skin color is dull with pale pink-yellow undertones; capillary refill is sluggish, greater than two seconds; cold extremities; denies chest pain.
Temperature: 99.2°F; denies having fever over the last few days
Nutritional/Fluid: Five feet ten inches, 165 pounds; denies having difficulty chewing or swallowing food or fluids, although he has not eaten food or drunk fluids today. He states, "I couldn't eat breakfast this morning. I felt sick." States he is experiencing nausea presently, however, denies vomiting. Skin is elastic with instant recoil.
Elimination: Denies difficulty with urination; voids five to seven times daily; reports last bowel movement was yesterday; normal bowel pattern is once every day or two. Foley catheter to gravity drainage, approximately 200 cc clear yellow urine is in the collection container; "When can I get this thing out? It's killing me!"
Rest/Sleep: Usually retires around 9:00 P.M. and sleeps until 5:00 A.M. Denies any difficulty sleeping.

Pain Avoidance: Rates headache as "seven" on scale of one to ten; the client points to the occipital region and states, "The pain is right here. Why won't it go away? They gave me some medicine in the emergency department. Can you give me another pill?" The client holds the back of his head. He describes the pain as constant, severe, and sharp.

Sexuality/Reproductive: Denies any concerns with sexual aspect of his life. "I don't feel like talking about that!"

Activity: States, "I don't get out much since my wife died two years ago. We used to go dancing. All I do now is just sit around the house. Sometimes my son picks me up and we go fishing." Upon arrival from the emergency department, the client was attempting to get up from the wheelchair and move to the hospital bed. He needed assistance moving his left leg. Left hand grip is reduced, left leg strength is reduced. "Why can't I move my leg and hand?"

Additional Data: The client answers all questions appropriately, denies any increased visual or hearing problems; pupils equal and reactive to light; able to blink eyes without difficulty, sclera pale pink, moist; skin is intact. IV is in his right forearm, D5 ½ NS infusing at 75 cc per hour; site is without redness or edema. He states he retired right before his wife died about two and one-half years ago and is comfortable in his retirement. Client is able to discuss the loss of wife without difficulty.

This scenario represents initial assessment data collected from the client's interview and physical assessment. The nurse utilizes a data collection format approved for his or her facility. As the nurse collects data, questions are asked to _____ or _____ data when necessary. The nurse is now ready to _____ the data, first by separating abnormal objective data (measurements and observations) from subjective data (statements and feelings that only the client can identify). Finally, the nurse _____ data to determine their relatedness and confirm that problems, risk problems, or strengths exist.

Subjective and Objective Data

Subjective Data

- Statement of headache for three days, rated as "seven" on scale of one to ten, described as constant, severe, sharp
- Nausea
- States weak left arm and left leg, "Can't move my arm or leg"
- Reports mild difficulty breathing
- States Foley catheter "is killing me"

Objective Data

- Blood pressure 152/84, temperature 99.2°F
- Right corner of mouth droops
- Difficulty pronouncing words
- Oxygen, two liters per nasal cannula
- Skin color dull, pale pink-yellow undertones, capillary refill sluggish greater than two seconds
- Foley catheter
- Holds occipital region of head
- Left grip and left leg with decreased strength
- Requires assistance to transfer from wheelchair to bed
- Decreased left pedal pulse
- Cold extremities

Clustering Data

Pain Avoidance	Oxygenation	Activity	Nutrition/Fluid Communication
• Headache for three days • Points to occipital region of head • Holds head • Requests for pain medications • Rates pain as "seven" on scale of one to ten, describes as sharp, continuous, severe • Blood pressure 152/84	• Reports mild difficulty breathing • Oxygen two liters via nasal cannula • Skin color dull, pale pink-yellow undertones, capillary refill greater than two seconds • Decreased pulse to left foot • Cold extremities	• Requires assistance with transfer from wheelchair to bed • Left hand and left leg weakness • Reports, "Can't move my leg and hand"	• Corner of right side of mouth droops • Difficulty pronouncing words • Has not eaten since symptoms began • Nausea

As you can see, objective and subjective data _____ and _____ each other. Once data are clustered, it becomes evident that problems and risk problems exist.

Use of _____ _____ would detect inconsistencies pertaining to the nutrition/fluid/communication category. Analysis reveals that data collection is incomplete. Has the client experienced a change in word pronunciation ability? Is facial drooping abnormal for the client? Data collected during observation and assessment conflict. Additional data must be collected before forming conclusions and planning care. For example, upon examination of a client who may be experiencing a cerebral vascular accident, one would expect facial and eye drooping to the affected side of the face, tearing of the affected eye, and possibly a change in pupillary response. The client may experience difficulty chewing or swallowing food and liquids. This information must be included for the nurse to have accurate and complete data for the next step of planning.

Mr. Norman was questioned regarding the above omissions to verify and validate data. He states, "I always have trouble pronouncing certain words, ever since I wrecked my motorcycle when I was in my early thirties. I injured a nerve in my face. My mouth droops a little, or at least it used to."

Assessment data are _____ using the approved format of the facility. The care plan will be developed from initial and ongoing data collection.

STEP 2: DIAGNOSIS

Diagnosis involves critical thought and judgment to _____, _____, and _____ assessment data. Problems, risk problems, and strengths are identified and labeled with NANDA nursing diagnoses. Once labeled, the nursing diagnosis communicates specific health care needs about the client to other members of the health care team involved in care.

The data collection tool used in the scenario provides information pertaining to specific areas of functioning: pain avoidance, oxygenation, activity, nutrition/fluid, and others. Review the list of clustered data under each category where actual problems are discovered during the assessment step. Information should be _____, _____, and _____.

The following is a list of actual or risk nursing diagnoses, related to, risk factors, and defining characteristics, which will be included in the care plan. Locate each nursing diagnosis in Appendix A and read the definition. Does the definition apply to Mr. Norman?

- *Pain, Acute*
  R/T: physical injuring agents, ineffective pain relief
  AEB: statement of headache for three days, rates pain as "seven" on scale of one to ten, requests for pain medication, blood pressure 152/84, holding head, points to occipital region when asked location of pain
- *Mobility, Impaired Physical*
  R/T: decreased muscle strength, neuromuscular impairment
  AEB: requires assistance with transfer from wheelchair to bed, left hand and left leg weakness, reports, "Can't move my leg and hand"
- *Tissue Perfusion, Altered (cerebral/peripheral)*
  R/T: interruption of arterial blood flow, pathology
  AEB: reports of mild dyspnea, skin color dull, pale pink-yellow undertones, capillary refill greater than two seconds, decreased pulse to left foot, cold extremities

Acute Pain and *Impaired Physical Mobility* are nursing diagnoses labeling *actual* client problems. The client may be *at risk* for problems related to nutrition and fluid balance resulting from nausea, if it should persist. Mr. Norman will be monitored for additional difficulties, such as impaired ability to carry out activities of daily living, feeding, grooming, and hygiene. If these or other problems become suspected or obvious, planning and development will begin. At this time, however, *no evidence* of additional problems or risk problems exists. *Do not read into the scenario.*

STEP 3: PLANNING AND OUTCOME IDENTIFICATION

Planning the care for the client involves several steps: identifying _____ _____ and _____, setting realistic _____ and _____ _____, determining nursing _____ and _____ _____, and finally, _____ and _____ the care plan. The planning step should involve discussing the plan with the client for input and collaboration. This encourages client participation and promotes the client's sense of control. Careful, effective planning advocates and ensures delivery of quality care.

Determining _____ involves analyzing data to discover situations requiring immediate attention. The client often communicates this during the _____ or _____. In Mr. Norman's case, pain or headache is the most outstanding problem. Several statements and requests were verbalized regarding pain medication. Consider Maslow's hierarchy of needs. The basic physiological needs include oxygenation, nutrition, hydration, elimination, body temperature maintenance, and pain avoidance.

In our scenario, Mr. Norman demonstrated outstanding signs and symptoms in areas of pain avoidance, oxygenation, and activity. After collaboration, he confirmed pain as the priority problem, at the moment.

Setting _____ and _____ _____ follow priority problem identification. *One* overall goal is determined for each nursing diagnosis. Goals are guidelines which help to individualize nursing interventions. Goals give _____ to the care plan and _____ on the _____ of the problem. *Goals* are general statements indicating the _____ or desired _____ in the client's health status, function, or behavior. *Expected outcomes* are stated in specific terms, describing methods through which the goal will be achieved.

Required components of goals include the _____ (client), _____, _____ of _____, and _____ _____. An optional component is the _____, referring to the aid which facilitates the performance. Goals and expected outcomes must be _____. Review the following goals/expected outcomes for Mr. Norman.

Can you identify each component of the goal statement?

Nursing diagnosis: Pain, Acute. R/T: physical injuring agents, ineffective pain relief. AEB: statement of headache for three days, rates pain as "seven" on scale of one to ten, requests for pain medication, blood pressure 152/84, holding head, points to occipital region when asked location of pain.

Goals/client outcomes: Mr. Norman will report pain relief to a minimal level within one hour after initiation of pain relief measures.

Nursing Diagnosis: Mobility, Impaired Physical. R/T: decreased muscle strength, neuromuscular impairment. AEB: requires assistance with transfer from wheelchair to bed, left hand and left leg weakness, reports, "Can't move my leg and hand"

Goals/client outcomes: Mr. Norman will demonstrate improved muscle strength by increasing physical activity with assistance of physical therapy prior to discharge.

Nursing diagnosis: Tissue Perfusion, Altered (cerebral/peripheral). R/T: interruption of arterial blood flow, pathology. AEB: reports of mild dyspnea, skin color dull, pale pink-yellow undertones, capillary refill greater than two seconds, decreased pulse to left foot, cold extremities.

Goals/client outcomes: Mr. Norman will demonstrate improved peripheral blood flow/perfusion within forty-eight hours of interventions.

Planning Nursing Interventions

Nursing interventions are activities _____ and _____ by the nursing team which benefit the client in a _____ manner. Interventions are selected based on scientific _____ and _____ of behavioral and physical sciences. Nurses use deliberate thought, decision making, and problem solving to determine actions which will aid in _____, _____, or _____ of the cause or etiology of the problem or nursing diagnosis. Nursing interventions are developed from the _____ of each nursing diagnosis. Generally, several interventions should be identified for each goal.

Interventions are selected based on the nurse's understanding of scientific principle and psychosocial or developmental theories. Understanding of the human body and mind allows for certain expected responses when interventions are carried out. The term *scientific rationale* is the _____ _____ for choosing a specific intervention. Scientific rationales are found in resource textbooks, such as medical-surgical or pediatric textbooks; references, such as pharmacology and clinical skills references; nursing and medical journals; and research articles. Another method of finding scientific rationales is to utilize one of the many nursing diagnosis or care plan resources available at most medical/nursing bookstores. Nursing interventions and scientific rationale for our scenario follow:

Nursing diagnosis: Pain, Acute. R/T: physical injuring agents, ineffective pain relief. AEB: statement of headache for three days, rates pain as "seven" on scale of one to ten, requests for pain medication, blood pressure 152/84, holding head, points to occipital region when asked location of pain.

Goals/client outcomes: Mr. Norman will report pain relief to a minimal level within one hour after initiation of pain relief measures.

Nursing Interventions and *Scientific Rationales*

1. Encourage client to report pain/discomfort location, intensity, duration, etc. using the pain scale. Obtain an exact description. *Changes in pain description may indicate a change in the client's condition.*
2. Administer smallest narcotic analgesic dose possible to aid in comfort, as per physician order. *Narcotic analgesics affect the level of consciousness and may interfere with neurological assessment.*

Nursing diagnosis: Mobility, Impaired Physical. R/T: decreased muscle strength, neuromuscular impairment. AEB: requires assistance with transfer from wheelchair to bed, left hand and left leg weakness, reports, "Can't move my leg and hand"

Goals/client outcomes: Mr. Norman will demonstrate improved muscle strength by increasing physical activity with assistance of physical therapy prior to discharge.

Nursing Interventions and *Scientific Rationales*

1. Monitor and screen client for mobility skills, such as bed mobility, unsupported sitting, standing and sitting down, transferring from bed to chair, and standing and

walking activities. *Screening and monitoring the client aids in identifying the level of impairment and provides a baseline of mobility abilities. Interventions may be planned appropriately.*

2. Consult with physical therapy for further evaluation and development of a mobility plan. *Allows staff to integrate collaborative plan which will enhance and maximize client's mobility.*

3. Perform passive range of motion to weakened extremities at least twice daily. Encourage active range of motion and assist when needed. *Strengthens muscles and prevents atrophy of muscle tissue.*

Nursing diagnosis: Tissue Perfusion, Altered (cerebral/peripheral). R/T: interruption of arterial blood flow, pathology. AEB: reports of mild dyspnea, skin color dull, pale pink-yellow undertones, capillary refill greater than two seconds, decreased pulse to left foot, cold extremities.

Goals/client outcomes: Mr. Norman will demonstrate improved peripheral blood flow/perfusion within forty-eight hours of interventions.

Nursing Interventions and *Scientific Rationales*

1. Monitor dorsalis pedis and posterior tibial pulses bilaterally for equal quality and rate. *Diminished or absent peripheral pulses indicate arterial insufficiency.*

2. Monitor for change in neurological status. Use neurological flow sheets to record results of neurological assessments. *Any change may indicate that the brain is deprived of adequate amount of oxygen due to further bleeding, increased intracranial pressure (ICP), or spasm of cerebral artery.*

3. Maintain extremities in dependent position and maintain physical rest. *To facilitate arterial blood flow through vessel narrowed by a thrombus.*

Once the plan of care is developed, it is shared with other members of the health care team involved in caring for the client. The plan is communicated verbally and through written documentation as the care plan. These actions promote continuity of care.

STEP 4: IMPLEMENTATION

During *implementation* planned nursing interventions are _____. This step begins with _____ and _____ of the client prior to initiating care. Each interaction with the client is an opportunity to _____, collect ongoing _____, and compare data to the client's _____. Nurses apply scientific knowledge and understanding, analytical skills, and deliberate thought to interpret ongoing data collection. Priority interventions are carried out first. However, nurses may _____ interventions for more than one problem at the same time.

STEP 5: EVALUATION

The *evaluation* phase measures the effectiveness of nursing care and the quality of care _____. However, evaluation, like assessment, is not a static activity, but _____ and _____, never ceasing. As interventions are carried out, client *responses* are evaluated and the client is reassessed. Questions are asked about the _____ and _____ of the intervention and the client's response to medical treatment, therapies, and nursing interventions. Are goals being met? If not, answers are sought to determine why.

Evaluation of the care plan focuses on changes in the client's health status, that is, if the client is progressing toward _____ _____. As the client's health status changes, the care plan is _____ to reflect the changing needs.

Lack of progress toward goal attainment may indicate the care plan needs _____ or _____. The nursing process sequence is _____ and _____ begins again. Collected data are analyzed, organized, and interpreted. All planning is compared to that previously determined, searching for _____ or _____. A new care plan is developed and executed.

During evaluation, when goals and expected outcomes are determined as having been achieved and the client no longer requires nursing assistance in this area, this portion of the care plan is _____. Nurses will continue to assess and evaluate the client for possible _____ of symptoms.

The completed care plan for Mr. Norman follows.

STUDENT PRACTICE

Instructions

Read the scenario and apply the five steps of the nursing process. Identify three appropriate nursing diagnoses (with *related to* and *as evidenced by* or *risk factors*). For each nursing diagnosis provide one goal/expected outcome, three nursing interventions with scientific rationale, and one evaluative statement. The care plan form is attached.

General Information

Information Provided by: client
Name: Mr. Paul Gonzales
Age: 57 years   **Sex:** male   **Race:** Hispanic
Admission Date/Time: December 14, 1999, 11:45 A.M.
Admitting Medical Diagnosis: alcohol withdrawal
Arrived on Unit by: wheelchair, from emergency department
Admitting Weight/Height/Vital Signs: temperature 99.8°F; pulse 112; respiration 24; blood pressure 168/92, weight 160 pounds, height five feet ten inches.
Client's Perception of Reason for Admission: client states, "I don't feel good."
Allergies: aspirin (ASA), penicillin (PCN)
Medications: no prescription medications, no over-the-counter medications, denies use of illegal medications

Assessment Data

Oxygenation: Denies difficulty breathing. Capillary refill greater than two seconds. Skin to extremities warm, dry. Respirations slightly increased. Cough, productive with tenacious, light brown, yellow sputum. Bilateral, midanterior lobes with rhonchi. Right midanterior lung with expiratory wheeze.

Temperature: Temperature 99.8°F; denies elevated temperature over last few days.

Nutritional/Fluid: States he usually eats one meal a day or snacks on peanuts and pretzels, "just to get something in my stomach." "I have all the nourishment I need, but it's liquid!" Poor oral hygiene; several dental caries and missing lower incisors. Oral mucosa pale. Conjunctiva pale pink. Skin turgor on forearm, inelastic. No nausea, no vomiting. Client states, "I have a burning sensation, here." Client points to epigastric abdominal region. "Just bring me some food. I'm hungry."

Elimination: Denies problems with bowel or bladder function. Voids without difficulty. Abdomen large, soft, nontender to palpation. Bowel sounds present in all four quadrants.

Sleep/Rest: Reports, "I can't sleep! That's one of my problems!" States he sometimes lies in bed for hours without sleep. "I've got too much on my mind."

Pain Avoidance: Reports discomfort in epigastric region. States, "It comes and goes. I don't need anything for it."

Sexuality/Reproductive: Married for thirty-three years to same wife. "I don't know how she puts up with me." Three grown children, two grandchildren.

Activity: Lives a fairly sedentary lifestyle. States, "I work in the office all day, go out with my friends, then come home and go to bed." No aerobic exercise. Hand tremors noted.

Additional Data: Refuses to talk about alcohol use/abuse. States he doesn't have a drinking problem. He reports he lost his job last week. "Now, I'll probably lose my wife and family." Mr. Gonzales is alert, answers questions appropriately, however, continuously turns to look over his shoulder. States, "I keep thinking I see bugs behind me. Keep them away!" He states, he sees "bugs" and "sometimes they're crawling on me." Eyes are wide and fearful when he describes the above. No visual deficit, no auditory deficit.

Nursing Diagnosis	Goal/Expected Outcomes	Nursing Intervention	Scientific Rationale	Evaluation
Pain. R/T: Physical injuring agents, ineffective pain relief. AEB: statement of headache for three days, rates pain as "seven" on scale of one to ten, requests for pain medication, blood pressure 152/84, holding head, points to occipital region when asked location of pain	Mr. Norman will report pain relief to a minimal level within one hour after initiation of pain relief measures.	1. Encourage client to report pain/discomfort location, intensity, duration, etc. using the pain scale. Obtain exact description. 2. Administer smallest narcotic analgesic dose possible to aid in comfort, as per physician order.	1. Changes in pain description may indicate a change in client's condition. 2. Narcotic analgesics affect the level of consciousness and may interfere with neurological assessment.	Client reports pain level reduced to "two" on scale of one to ten.
Mobility, Impaired Physical. R/T: decreased muscle strength, neuromuscular impairment AEB: requires assistance with transfer from wheelchair to bed, left hand and left leg weakness, reports, "Can't move my leg and hand"	Mr. Norman will demonstrate improved muscle strength by increasing physical activity with assistance of physical therapy prior to discharge.	1. Monitor and screen client for mobility skills, such as bed mobility, unsupported sitting, standing, and sitting down, transferring from bed to chair, and standing and walking activities. 2. Consult with physical therapy for further evaluation and development of a mobility plan. 3. Perform passive range of motion to weakened extremities at least twice daily. Encourage active range of motion and assist when needed.	1. Screening and monitoring the client aids in identification of level of impairment and provides a baseline of mobility abilities. Interventions may be planned appropriately. Allows staff to integrate collaborative plan which will enhance and maximize client's mobility. 2. 3. Strengthens muscles and prevents atrophy of muscle tissue.	Client performs limited active range of motion to left hand and leg, assists in passive range of motion twice daily.
Tissue Perfusion, Altered (cerebral/peripheral) R/T: interruption of arterial blood flow, pathology. AEB: reports of mild dyspnea, skin color dull, pale pink-yellow undertones, capillary refill greater than two seconds, decreased pulse to left foot, cold extremities.	Mr. Norman will demonstrate improved peripheral blood flow/perfusion within forty-eight hours of interventions.	1. Monitor dorsalis pedis and posterior tibial pulses bilaterally for equal quality and rate. 2. Monitor for change in neurological status. Use neurological flow sheets to record results of neurological assessments. 3. Maintain extremities in dependent position and maintain physical rest.	1. Diminished or absent peripheral pulses indicate arterial insufficiency. 2. Any change may indicate that the brain is deprived of adequate amount of oxygen due to further bleeding, increased intracranial pressure (ICP), or spasm of cerebral artery. 3. To facilitate arterial blood flow through vessel narrowed by a thrombus.	Feet warm to touch, capillary refill greater than two seconds; no dyspnea

FIGURE 7:1 Documented Care Plan for Tom Norman

Appendix A

1999–2000 NORTH AMERICAN NURSING DIAGNOSIS ASSOCIATION (NANDA): Diagnoses, Definitions, Risk Factors or Related Factors, and Defining Characteristics

Reprinted with permission of North American Nursing Diagnosis Association, 1999, Philadelphia: NANDA.

Activity intolerance

Definition: a state in which an individual has insufficient physiological or psychological energy to endure or complete required or desired daily activities

Related factors: bedrest or immobility; generalized weakness; imbalance between oxygen supply/demand; sedentary lifestyle

Defining characteristics: verbal report of fatigue or weakness; abnormal heart rate or blood pressure response to activity; electrocardiographic changes reflecting arrhythmias or ischemia; exertional discomfort or dyspnea

Activity intolerance, risk for

Definition: a state in which an individual is at risk of experiencing insufficient physiological or psychological energy to endure or complete required or desired daily activities

Risk factors: inexperience with the activity; presence of circulatory/respiratory problems; history of previous intolerance; deconditioned status

Adaptive capacity, intracranial, decreased

Definition: a clinical state in which intracranial fluid dynamic mechanisms that normally compensate for increases in intracranial volumes are compromised, resulting in repeated, disproportionate increases in intracranial pressure in response to a variety of noxious and non-noxious stimuli

Related factors: decreased cerebral perfusion pressure $\leq$50–60 mm Hg; sustained increase in ICP $\geq$ 10–15 mm Hg; systemic hypotension with intracranial hypertension; brain injuries

Defining characteristics: repeated increases of greater than 10 mm Hg for more than 5 minutes following any of a variety of external stimuli; baseline ICP equal to or greater than 10 mm Hg; disproportionate increase in ICP following single environmental or nursing maneuver stimulus; elevated P_2 ICP waveform; volume pressure response test variation (volume-pressure ratio >2, pressure-volume index <10); wide amplitude ICP waveform

Adjustment, impaired

Definition: inability to modify life style/behavior in a manner consistent with a change in health status

Related factors: low state of optimism; intense emotional state; negative attitudes toward health behavior; failure to intend to change behavior; multiple stressors; absence of social support for changed beliefs and practices; disability or health status change requiring change in life style; lack of motivation to change behaviors

Defining characteristics: denial of health status change; failure to achieve optimal sense of control; failure to take actions that would prevent further health problems; demonstration of non-acceptance of health status change

Airway clearance, ineffective

Definition: inability to clear secretions or obstructions from the respiratory tract to maintain a clear airway

Related factors:

Environmental: smoking; smoke inhalation; second-hand smoke

Obstructed airway: airway spasm; retained secretions; excessive mucus; presence of artificial airway; foreign body in airway; secretions in the bronchi; exudate in the alveoli

Physiological: neuromuscular dysfunction; hyperplasia of the bronchial walls; chronic obstructive pulmonary disease; infection; asthma; allergic airways, trauma

Defining characteristics: dyspnea; diminished breath sounds; orthopnea; adventitious breath sounds (rales, crackles, rhonchi; wheezes); ineffective or absent cough; sputum; cyanosis; difficulty vocalizing; wide-eyed [look]; changes in respiratory rate and rhythm; restlessness

Anxiety

Definition: a vague, uneasy feeling of discomfort or dread accompanied by an autonomic response; the source is often nonspecific or unknown to the individual; a feeling of apprehension caused by anticipation of danger. It is an altering signal that warns of impending danger and enables the individual to take measures to deal with threat

Related factors: exposure to toxins; threat to or change in role status; unconscious conflict about essential goals/values of life; familial association/heredity; unmet needs; interpersonal crises; threat of death; threat to or change in health status; threat to or change in interaction patterns; threat to or change in role function; threat to self-concept; unconscious conflict abut essential values/goals of life; threat to or change in environment; stress; threat to change in economic status; substance abuse

Defining characteristics:

Behavioral: diminished productivity; scanning and vigilance; poor eye contact; restlessness; glancing about; extraneous movement (e.g., foot shuffling, hand/arm movements); expressed concerns due to change in life events; insomnia; fidgeting

Affective: regretful; irritability; anguish; scared; jittery; overexcited; painful and persistent increased helplessness; rattled; uncertainty; increased wariness; focus on self; feelings of inadequacy; fearful; distressed; apprehension; anxious

Physiological: voice quivering, trembling/hand tremors; insomnia; shakiness

Parasympathetic: abdominal pain; decreased blood pressure; decreased pulse; diarrhea; faintness; fatigue; nausea; sleep disturbance; urinary urgency; urinary hesitancy; urinary frequency; tingling in extremities

Sympathetic: anorexia; dry mouth; increased respiration; increased blood pressure; increased pulse; increased tension; increased reflexes; increased perspiration; cardiovascular excitation; facial tension; heart pounding; pupil dilation; respiratory difficulties; superficial vasoconstriction; weakness; twitching

Cognitive: blocking of thought; confusion; preoccupation; forgetfulness; rumination; impaired attention; decreased perceptual field; fear of unspecific consequences; tendency to blame others; difficulty concentrating; diminished ability to problem solve; diminished learning ability; awareness of physiologic symptoms

Anxiety, death

Definition: the apprehension, worry, or fear related to death or dying

Related factors: to be developed

Defining characteristics: worrying about the impact of one's own death on significant others; powerless over issues related to dying; fear of loss of physical and/or mental abilities when dying; anticipated pain related to dying; deep sadness; fear of the process of dying; concerns of overworking the caregiver as terminal illness incapacitates self; concern about meeting one's creator or feeling doubtful about the existence of a god or higher being; total loss of control over any aspect of one's own death; negative death images or unpleasant thoughts about any event related to death or dying; fear of delayed demise; fear of premature death because it prevents the accomplishment of important life goals; worrying about being the cause of other's grief and suffering; fear of leaving family alone after death; fear of developing a terminal illness; denial of one's own mortality or impending death

Aspiration, risk for
Definition: the state in which an individual is at risk for entry of gastrointestinal secretions, oropharyngeal secretions, or solids or fluids into tracheobronchial passages
Risk factors: increased intragastric pressure; tube feedings; situations hindering elevation of upper body; reduced level of consciousness; presence of tracheostomy or endotracheal tube; medication administration; wired jaws; increased gastric residual; incomplete lower esophageal sphincter; impaired swallowing; gastrointestinal tubes; facial, oral, neck surgery or trauma; depressed cough and gag reflexes; decreased gastrointestinal motility; delayed gastric emptying

Body image disturbance
Definition: confusion in mental picture of one's physical self
Related factors: psychosocial; biophysical; cognitive/perceptual; cultural or spiritual; developmental changes; illness; trauma or injury; surgery; illness treatment
Defining characteristics: nonverbal response to actual or perceived change in structure and/or function; verbalization of feelings that reflect an altered view of one's body in appearance, structure, or function; verbalization of perceptions that reflect an altered view of one's body in appearance, structure, or function; behaviors of avoidance, monitoring, or acknowledgment of one's body
Objective: missing body part; trauma to nonfunctioning part; not touching body part; hiding or overexposing body part (intentional or unintentional); actual change in [body] structure and/or function; change in social involvement; change in ability to estimate spatial relationship of body to environment; extension of body boundary to incorporate environmental objects; not looking at body part
Subjective: refusal to verify actual change; preoccupation with change or loss; personalization of part or loss by name; depersonalization of [body] part or loss by impersonal pronouns; negative feelings about body (e.g., feelings of helplessness, hopelessness, or powerlessness); verbalization of change in lifestyle; focus on past strength, function, or appearance; fear of rejection or of reaction by others; emphasis on remaining strengths and heightened achievement

Body temperature, altered, risk for
Definition: the state in which an individual is at risk for failure to maintain body temperature within normal range.
Risk factors: altered metabolic rate; illness or trauma affecting temperature regulation; medications causing vasoconstriction or vasodilation; inappropriate clothing for environmental temperature; inactivity or vigorous activity; extremes of weight; extremes of ages; dehydration; sedation; exposure to cold/cool or warm/hot environments.

Breastfeeding, effective
Definition: the state in which a mother-infant dyad/family exhibits adequate proficiency and satisfaction with breastfeeding process
Related factors: infant gestational age greater than 34 weeks; supportive source; normal infant oral structure; maternal confidence; basic breastfeeding knowledge; normal breast structure
Defining characteristics: effective mother/infant communication patterns; regular and sustained suckling/swallowing at the breast; appropriate infant weight pattern for age; infant is content after feeding; mother able to position infant at breast to promote a successful latch-on response; signs and/or symptoms of oxytocin release; adequate infant elimination patterns for age; eagerness of infant to nurse; maternal verbalization of satisfaction with the breastfeeding process

Breastfeeding, ineffective
Definition: the state in which a mother, infant, or child experiences dissatisfaction or difficulty with the breastfeeding process
Related factors: nonsupportive partner/family; previous breast surgery; infant receiving supplemental feedings with artificial nipple; prematurity; previous history of breastfeeding failure; poor infant sucking reflex; maternal breast anomaly; maternal anxiety or ambivalence; interruption in breastfeeding; infant anomaly; knowledge deficit
Defining characteristics: unsatisfactory breastfeeding process; nonsustained suckling at the breast; resisting latching on; unresponsive to other comfort measures; persistence of sore nipples beyond the first week of breastfeeding; observable

signs of inadequate infant intake; insufficient emptying of each breast per feeding; infant inability to attach on to maternal breast correctly; infant arching and crying at the breast; infant exhibiting fussiness and crying within the first hour after breastfeeding; actual or perceived inadequate milk supply; no observable signs of oxytocin release; insufficient opportunity for suckling at the breast

Breastfeeding, interrupted

Definition: a break in the continuity of the breastfeeding process as a result of inability or inadvisability to put baby to breast for feeding

Related factors: contraindications to breastfeeding; maternal employment; maternal or infant illness; need to abruptly wean infant; prematurity

Defining characteristics: infant does not receive nourishment at the breast for some or all of feedings; lack of knowledge regarding expression and storage of breastmilk; maternal desire to maintain lactation and provide (or eventually provide) her breastmilk for her infant's nutritional needs; separation of mother and infant

Breathing pattern, ineffective

Definition: inspiration and/or expiration that does not provide adequate ventilation

Related factors: hyperventilation; hypoventilation syndrome; bony deformity; pain; chest wall deformity; anxiety; decreased energy/fatigue; neuromuscular dysfunction; musculoskeletal impairment; perception/cognitive impairment; obesity; spinal cord injury; body position; neurological immaturity; respiratory muscle fatigue

Defining characteristics: decreased inspiratory/expiratory pressure; decreased minute ventilation; use of accessory muscles to breathe; nasal flaring; dyspnea; altered chest excursion; shortness of breath; assumption of three-point position; pursed lip breathing; prolonged expiration phases; increased anterior-posterior diameter; respiratory rate (infants: age 0–12 mo <25 or >60; children: 1–4 yr <20 or >30; children: 5–14 yr <15 or >25; adults: [age 14 or older] <11 or >24); depth of breathing (adults V_T 500 ml at rest, infants 6–8 ml/kg); timing ratio; orthopnea; decreased vital capacity

Cardiac output, decreased

Definition: a state in which the blood pumped by the heart is inadequate to meet the metabolic demands of the body

Related factors: to be developed; [possible non-NANDA factors: cardiac anomaly (specify); impaired electrical conduction; dysrhythmia; hypovolemia]

Defining characteristics: fatigue; variations in blood pressure readings; restlessness; rales; orthopnea/paroxysmal nocturnal dyspnea; jugular vein distention; dyspnea; decreased peripheral pulses; cold, clammy skin; arrhythmias; oliguria; edema; skin color changes; chest pain; weight gain; wheezing; elevated pulmonary artery pressures; increased respiratory rate; use of accessory muscles; ECG changes; ejection fraction <40%; abnormal chest x-ray (pulmonary vascular congestion); abnormal cardiac enzymes; altered mental states; decreased peripheral pulses; decreased cardiac output by thermodilution method; increased heart rate; S_3 and S_4 (gallop rhythm); cough; mixed venous oxygen (SaO_2)

Caregiver role strain

Definition: a caregiver's felt or exhibited difficulty in performing a family caregiver role

Related factors:

Resources: caregiver is not developmentally ready for caregiver role; lack of respite resources; lack of support from significant others; lack of recreational resources; insufficient information; inadequate transportation; insufficient finances; inadequate equipment for providing care; inadequate community services

Roles and relationships: history of family dysfunction; unrealistic expectations of caregiver by care receiver; change in relationship; history of marginal family coping

Social: alienation from family, friends, and coworkers; insufficient recreation

Individual: instability of care receiver's health; problem behaviors; psychological or cognitive problems in care receiver; illness chronicity

Caregiver: ongoing changes in activities; psychological or cognitive problems; addiction or codependency; unrealistic expectations of self; marginal caregiver's coping patterns; unpredictability of care situation; amount of activities; 24 hour care responsibility; inability to fulfill one's own or other's expectations

Situational: inadequate physical environment for providing care (e.g., housing, transportation, community services, equipment); inexperience with caregiving; presence of abuse or violence; family/caregiver isolation; caregiver's competing role commitments; complexity/amount of caregiving tasks

Physiological: increasing care needs and/or dependency; unpredictable illness course or instability in the care receiver's health; illness severity of the care receiver, addiction or codependency of care receiver; discharge of family member with significant home care needs; caregiver health impairment

Defining characteristics: apprehension about possible institutionalization of care receiver; apprehension about the future regarding care receiver's health and the caregiver's ability to provide care; difficulty performing required activities; apprehension about receiver's care when caregiver is ill or deceased; inability to complete caregiving tasks; preoccupation with care routine; altered caregiving activities; altered caregiver health status (e.g., hypertension, cardiovascular disease, diabetes, headaches, gastrointestinal upset, weight change, rash)

Caregiver role strain, risk for

Definition: a caregiver is vulnerable for felt difficulty in performing the family caregiver role

Risk factors: caregiver is not developmentally ready for caregiver role (e.g., a young adult needing to provide care for middle-aged); inadequate physical environment for providing care (e.g., housing, transportation, community services, equipment); unpredictable illness course or instability in the care receiver's health; psychological or cognitive problems in care receiver; presence of situational stressors which normally affect families (e.g., significant loss, disaster or crisis, economic vulnerability, major life events); presence of abuse or violence; premature birth/congenital defect; past history of poor relationship between caregiver and care receiver; marginal family adaptation or dysfunction prior to the caregiving situation; marginal caregiver's coping patterns; lack of respite and recreation for caregiver; inexperience with caregiving; caregiver is female; addiction or codependency; care receiver exhibits deviant, bizarre behavior; caregiver's competing role commitments; caregiver health impairment; illness severity of the care receiver; caregiver is spouse; complexity/amount of caregiving tasks; developmental delay or retardation of the care receiver or caregiver; discharge of family member with significant home care needs; duration of caregiving required; family/caregiver isolation

Communication, impaired verbal

Definition: the state in which an individual experiences a decreased, delayed, or absent ability to receive, process, transmit, and use a system of symbols; anything that has meaning (i.e., transmits meaning)

Related factors: decrease in circulation to brain; cultural difference; psychological barriers (e.g., psychosis, lack of stimuli); physical barrier (e.g., tracheostomy, intubation); anatomical defect (e.g., cleft palate, alteration of the neuromuscular visual system, auditory system, or phonatory apparatus); brain tumor; differences related to developmental age; side-effects of medication; environmental barriers; absence of significant others; altered perceptions; lack of information; stress; alteration of self-esteem or self-concept; physiological conditions; alteration of central nervous system; weakening of the musculoskeletal system; emotional conditions.

Defining characteristics: willful refusal to speak; disorientation in the three spheres of time, space, person; unable to speak dominant language; does not or cannot speak; speaks or verbalizes with difficulty; inappropriate verbalization; difficulty forming words or sentences (e.g., aphonia, dyslalia, dysarthria); stuttering; slurring; difficulty expressing thought verbally (e.g., aphasia, dysphasia apraxia, dyslexia); dyspnea; absence of eye contact or difficulty in selective attending; difficulty in comprehending and maintaining the usual communication pattern; partial or total visual deficit; inability or difficulty in use of facial or body expressions.

Confusion, acute

Definition: the abrupt onset of a cluster of global, transient changes and disturbances in attention, cognition, psychomotor activity, level of consciousness, and/or sleep/wake cycle

Related factors: over 60 years of age; alcohol abuse; delirium; dementia; drug abuse

Defining characteristics: lack of motivation to initiate and/or follow through with goal-directed or purposeful behavior; fluctuation in psychomotor activity; misperceptions; fluctuation in cognition; increased agitation or restlessness; fluctuation in level of consciousness; fluctuation in sleep-wake cycle; hallucinations

Confusion, chronic

Definition: an irreversible, long-standing and/or progressive deterioration of intellect and personality characterized by decreased ability to interpret environmental stimuli, decreased capacity for intellectual thought processes and manifested by disturbances of memory, orientation, and behavior

Related factors: multi-infarct dementia; Korsakoff's psychosis; head injury; Alzheimer's disease; cerebral vascular accident

Defining characteristics: altered interpretation/response to stimuli; clinical evidence of organic impairment; progressive/long-standing cognitive impairment; altered personality; impaired memory (short-term and long-term); impaired socialization, no change in level of consciousness

Constipation

Definition: a decrease in a person's normal frequency of defecation accompanied by difficult or incomplete passage of stool and/or passage of excessively hard, dry stool
Related factors:
Functional: recent environmental changes; habitual denial/ignoring of urge to defecate; insufficient physical activity; irregular defecation habits; inadequate toileting (e.g., timeliness, positioning for defecation, privacy); abdominal muscle weakness
Psychological: depression; emotional stress; mental confusion
Pharmacological: antilipemic agents; laxative overdose; calcium carbonate; aluminum-containing antacids; nonsteroidal anti-inflammatory agents; opiates; anticholinergics; diuretics; iron salts; phenothiazides; sedatives; sympathomimetics; bismuth salts; antidepressants; calcium channel blockers
Mechanical: rectal abscess or ulcer; pregnancy; rectal anal fissures; tumors; megacolon (Hirschsprung's disease); electrolyte imbalance; rectal prolapse; prostate enlargement; neurological impairment; rectal anal stricture; rectocele; postsurgical obstruction; hemorrhoids; obesity
Physiological: poor eating habits; decreased motility of gastrointestinal tract; inadequate dentition or oral hygiene; insufficient fiber intake; insufficient fluid intake; change in usual foods and eating patterns; dehydration

Constipation, perceived

Definition: the state in which an individual makes a self-diagnosis of constipation and ensures a daily bowel movement through the use of laxatives, enemas, and suppositories
Related factors: impaired thought processes; faulty appraisal; cultural/family health beliefs
Defining characteristics: expectation of a daily bowel movement with the resulting overuse of laxatives, enemas, and suppositories; expected passage of stool at same time every day

Constipation, risk for

Definition: at risk for a decrease in a person's normal frequency of defecation accompanied by difficult or incomplete passage of stool and/or passage of excessively hard, dry stool
Risk factors:
Functional: habitual denial/ignoring of urge to defecate; recent environmental changes; inadequate toileting (e.g., timeliness, positioning for defecation, privacy); irregular defecation habits; insufficient physical activity; abdominal muscle weakness
Psychological: emotional stress; mental confusion; depression
Physiological: insufficient fiber intake; dehydration; inadequate dentition or oral hygiene; poor eating habits; insufficient fluid intake; change in usual foods and eating patterns; decreased motility of gastrointestinal tract
Pharmacological: Phenothiazides, nonsteroidal anti-inflammatory agents; sedatives; aluminum-containing antacids; laxative overuse; iron salts; anticholinergics; antidepressants; anticonvulsants; antilipemic agents; calcium channel blockers; calcium carbonate; diuretics; sympathomimetics; opiates; bismuth salts
Mechanical: rectal abscess or ulcer; pregnancy; rectal anal stricture; postsurgical obstruction; rectal anal fissures; megacolon (Hirschsprung's disease); electrolyte imbalance; tumors; prostate enlargement; rectocele; rectal prolapse; neurological impairment; hemorrhoids; obesity

Coping, defensive

Definition: the state in which an individual repeatedly projects falsely positive self-evaluation based on a self-protective pattern that defends against underlying perceived threats to positive self-regard
Related factors: to be developed; possible non-NANDA factors: situational crisis (specify); physical illness (specify); psychologic impairment (specify)
Defining characteristics: grandiosity; rationalizes failures; hypersensitive to slight/criticism; denial of obvious problems/weaknesses; projection of blame/responsibility; lack of follow through or participation in treatment or therapy; su-

perior attitude toward others; hostile laughter or ridicule of others; difficulty in reality-testing perceptions; difficulty establishing/maintaining relationships

Coping, ineffective community

Definition: a pattern of community activities for adaptation and problem solving that is unsatisfactory for meeting the demands or needs of the community

Related factors: natural or man-made disasters; ineffective or nonexistent community systems (e.g., lack of emergency medical system, transportation system, or disaster planning systems); deficits in community social support services and resources; inadequate resources for problem solving

Defining characteristics: expressed community powerlessness; deficits in community participation; excessive community conflicts; expressed vulnerability; high illness rates; stressors perceived as excessive; community does not meet its own expectations; increased social problems (e.g., homicides, vandalism, arson, terrorism, robbery, infanticide, abuse, divorce, unemployment, poverty, militancy, mental illness)

Coping, potential for enhanced community

Definition: a pattern of community activities for adaptation and problem solving that is satisfactory for meeting the demands or needs of the community but can be improved for management of current and future problems/stressors

Related factors: community has a sense of power to manage stressors; social supports available; resources available for problem solving

Defining characteristics: deficits in one or more characteristics that indicate effective coping; positive communication between community/aggregates and larger community; programs for recreation and relaxation; resources sufficient for managing stressors; agreement that community is responsible for stress management; active planning by community for predicted stressors; active problem solving by community when faced with issues; positive communication among community members

Coping: disabling, ineffective family

Definition: behavior of significant person (family member or other primary person) that disables his/her capacities and the client's capacities to effectively address tasks essential to either person's adaptation to the health challenge

Related factors: significant person with chronically unexpressed feelings of guilt, anxiety, hostility, despair, etc., arbitrary handling of family's resistance to treatment, which tends to solidify defensiveness as it fails to deal adequately with underlying anxiety; dissonant discrepancy of coping styles for dealing with adaptive tasks by the significant person and client or among significant people; highly ambivalent family relationships

Defining characteristics: intolerance; agitation; depression; aggression; hostility; taking on illness signs of client; rejection; psychosomaticism; neglectful care of the client in regard to basic human needs and/or illness treatment; impaired restructuring of a meaningful life for self; impaired individualization; prolonged over-concern for client; distortion of reality regarding the client's health problem, including extreme denial about its existence or severity; desertion; decisions and actions by family that are detrimental to economic or social well-being; carrying on usual routines, disregarding client's needs; abandonment; client's development of helplessness, inactive dependence; disregarding needs

Coping: compromised, ineffective family

Definition: a usually supportive primary person (family member or close friend) is providing insufficient, ineffective or compromised support, comfort, assistance or encouragement which may be needed by the client to manage or master adaptive tasks related to his/her health challenge

Related factors: temporary preoccupation by a significant person who is trying to manage emotional conflicts and personal suffering and is unable to perceive or act effectively in regard to client's needs; temporary family disorganization and role changes; prolonged disease or disability progression that exhausts supportive capacity of significant people; other situational or developmental crises or situations the significant person may be facing; inadequate or incorrect information or understanding by a primary person; little support provided by client, in turn, for primary person

Defining characteristics:

Objective: significant person attempts assistive or supportive behaviors with less than satisfactory results; significant person displays protective behavior disproportionate (too little or too much) to the client's abilities or need for autonomy; significant person withdraws or enters into limited or temporary personal communication with the client at the time of need

Subjective: client expresses or confirms a concern or complaint about significant other's response to his or her health problem; significant person describes or confirms an inadequate understanding or knowledge base, which interferes with effective assistive or supportive behaviors; significant person describes preoccupation with personal reaction (e.g., fear, anticipatory grief, guilt, anxiety) to client's illness, disability, or other situational or developmental crises

Coping, family: potential for growth

Definition: effective managing of adaptive tasks by family member involved with the client's health challenge, who now is exhibiting desire and readiness for enhanced health and growth in regard to self and in relation to the client
Related factors: needs sufficiently gratified and adaptive tasks effectively addressed to enable goals of self-actualization to surface
Defining characteristics: individual expressing interest in making contact on a one-to-one basis or on a mutual-aid group basis with another person who has experienced a similar situation; family member moving in direction of health promoting and enriching life-style that supports and monitors maturational processes, audits and negotiates treatment programs, and chooses experiences that optimize wellness; family member attempting to describe growth impact of crisis on his or her own values, priorities, goal, or relationships

Coping, individual, ineffective

Definition: inability to form a valid appraisal of the stressors, inadequate choices of practiced responses, and/or inability to use available resources
Related factors: gender differences in coping strategies; inadequate level of confidence in ability to cope; uncertainty; inadequate social support created by characteristics of relationships; inadequate level of perception of control; inadequate resources available; high degree of threat; situational or maturational crises; disturbance in pattern of tension release; inadequate opportunity to prepare for stressor; inability to conserve adaptive energies; disturbance in pattern of appraisal of threat
Defining characteristics: lack of goal-directed behavior/resolution of problems including inability to attend and difficulty with organizing information; sleep disturbance; abuse of chemical agents; decreased use of social support; use of forms of coping that impede adaptive behavior; poor concentration; inadequate problem solving; verbalization of inability to cope or inability to ask for help; inability to meet basic needs; destructive behavior toward self or others; inability to meet role expectations; high illness rate; change in usual communication patterns; fatigue; risk taking

Decisional conflict (specify)

Definition: the state of uncertainty about course of action to be taken when choice among competing actions involves risk, loss, or challenge to personal life values
Related factors: support system deficit; perceived threat to value system; multiple or divergent sources of information; lack of relevant information; unclear personal values/beliefs; lack of experience or interference with decision making
Defining characteristics: verbalization of undesired consequences of alternative actions being considered; verbalized uncertainty about choices; vacillation between alternative choices; delayed decision making; verbalized feeling of distress while attempting a decision; self-focusing; physical signs of distress or tension (e.g., increased heart rate, increased muscle tension, restlessness); questioning personal values and beliefs while attempting a decision

Denial, ineffective

Definition: the state of a conscious or unconscious attempt to disavow the knowledge or meaning of an event to reduce anxiety/fear to the detriment of health
Related factors: to be developed
Defining characteristics: delays seeking or refuses health care attention to the detriment of health; does not perceive personal relevance of symptoms or danger; displaces source of symptoms to other organs; displays inappropriate affect; does not admit fear of death or invalidism; makes dismissive gestures or comments when speaking of distressing events; minimizes symptoms; unable to admit impact of disease on life pattern; uses home remedies (self-treatment) to relieve symptoms; displaces fear of impact of the condition

Dentition, altered
Definition: disruption in tooth development/eruption patterns or structural integrity of individual teeth
Related factors: ineffective oral hygiene; sensitivity to heat or cold; barriers to self-care; access or economic barriers to professional care; nutritional deficits; dietary habits; genetic predisposition; selected prescription medications; premature loss of primary teeth; excessive intake of fluorides; chronic vomiting; chronic use of tobacco, coffee, tea, or red wine; lack of knowledge regarding dental health; excessive use of abrasive cleaning agents; bruxism
Defining characteristics: excessive plaque; crown or root caries; halitosis; tooth enamel discoloration; toothache; loose teeth; excessive calculus; incomplete eruption for age (may be primary or permanent teeth); malocclusion or tooth misalignment; premature loss of primary teeth; worn down or abraded teeth; tooth fracture(s); missing teeth or complete absence; erosion of enamel; asymmetrical facial expression

Development, risk for altered
Definition: at risk for delay of 25% or more in one or more of the areas of social or self-regulatory behavior, or cognitive, language, gross or fine motor skills
Risk factors:
Prenatal: maternal age <15 or (sic <) >35 years; substance abuse; infections; genetic or endocrine disorders; unplanned or unwanted pregnancy; lack of, late, or poor prenatal care; inadequate nutrition; illiteracy; poverty
Individual: prematurity; seizures; congenital or genetic disorders; positive drug screening test; brain damage (e.g., hemorrhage in postnatal period, shaken baby, abuse, accident); vision impairment; hearing impairment or frequent otitis media; chronic illness; technology-dependent; failure to thrive, inadequate nutrition; foster or adopted child; lead poisoning; chemotherapy; radiation therapy; natural disaster; behavior disorders; substance abuse
Environmental: poverty; violence
Caregiver: abuse; mental illness; mental retardation or severe learning disability

Diarrhea
Definition: passage of loose, unformed stools
Related factors:
Psychological: high stress levels and anxiety
Situational: alcohol abuse; toxins; laxative abuse; radiation; tube feedings; adverse effects of medications; contaminants; travel
Physiological: inflammation; malabsorption; infectious processes; irritation; parasites
Defining characteristics: hyperactive bowel sounds; at least 3 loose liquid stools per day; urgency; abdominal pain; cramping

Disuse syndrome, risk for
Definition: a state in which an individual is at risk for deterioration of body systems as the result of prescribed or unavoidable musculoskeletal inactivity; complications from immobility can include pressure ulcer, constipation, stasis of pulmonary secretions, thrombosis, urinary tract infection/retention, decreased strength/endurance, orthostatic hypotension, decreased range of joint motion, disorientation, body image disturbance and powerlessness.
Risk factors: severe pain; mechanical immobilization; altered level of consciousness; prescribed immobilization; paralysis

Diversional activity deficit
Definition: the state in which an individual experiences decreased stimulation from or decreased interest or engagement in recreational or leisure activities
Related factors: environmental lack of diversional activity as in long-term hospitalization; frequent, lengthy treatments
Defining characteristics: usual hobbies cannot be undertaken in hospital; patient's statements regarding: boredom, wish there was something to do, to read, etc.

Dysreflexia
Definition: the state in which an individual with a spinal cord injury at T7 or above experiences a life threatening uninhibited sympathetic response of the nervous system to a noxious stimulus
Related factors: bladder distention; bowel distention; lack of patient and care-giver knowledge; skin irritation

Defining characteristics: pallor (below the injury); paroxysmal hypertension (sudden periodic elevated blood pressure where systolic pressure is over 140 mm Hg and diastolic is above 90 mm Hg); red splotches on skin (above the injury); bradycardia or tachycardia (pulse rate of less than 60 or over 100 beats per minute); diaphoresis (above the injury); headache (a diffuse pain in different portions of the head and not confined to any nerve distribution area); blurred vision; chest pain; chills; conjunctival congestion; Horner's syndrome (contraction of the pupil, partial ptosis of the eyelid, enophthalmos and sometimes loss of sweating over the affected side of the face); metallic taste in mouth; nasal congestion; paresthesia; pilomotor reflex (gooseflesh formation when skin is cooled)

Dysreflexia, risk for autonomic

Definition: a lifelong threatening uninhibited response of the sympathetic nervous system for an individual with a spinal cord injury or lesion at T8 or above, and having recovered from spinal shock
Risk factors:
Cardiac/Pulmonary problems: pulmonary emboli
Gastrointestinal problems: distention; constipation; enemas; stimulation (e.g., digital, instrumentation, surgery); gastrointestinal system pathology; gastric ulcers; esophageal reflux
Neurological problems: painful or irritating stimuli below the level of injury
Regulatory problems: temperature fluctuations
Reproductive problems: menstruation; sexual intercourse; ejaculation
Integumentary problems: cutaneous stimulations (e.g., pressure ulcer, ingrown toenail, dressings, burns, rash); heterotrophic bone
Situational problems: positioning; range of motion exercises; pregnancy; labor and delivery; drug reactions (e.g., decongestants, sympathomimetics, vasoconstrictors, narcotic withdrawal); constrictive clothing; fractures; deep vein thrombosis; ovarian cyst; surgical procedures
Urological problems: bladder distention; spasm; instrumentation; epididymitis; urethritis; infection

Energy field disturbance

Definition: a disruption of the flow of energy surrounding a person's being that results in disharmony of the body, mind, and/or spirit
Related factors: to be developed
Defining characteristics: movement (wave/spike/tingling/dense/flowing); sounds (tone/words); temperature change (warmth/coolness); visual changes (image/color); disruption of the field (vacant/hold/spike/bulge)

Environmental interpretation syndrome, impaired

Definition: consistent lack of orientation to person, place, time, or circumstances over more than three to six months, necessitating a protective environment
Related factors: depression; Huntington's disease; dementia (e.g., Alzheimer's, multi-infarct dementia, Pick's disease, AIDS dementia, alcoholism, Parkinson's disease)
Defining characteristics: chronic confusional states; consistent disorientation in known and unknown environments; loss of occupation or social functioning from memory decline; slow in responding to questions; inability to follow simple directions, instructions; inability to concentrate; inability to reason

Failure to thrive, adult

Definition: a progressive functional deterioration of a physical and cognitive nature; the individual's ability to live with multisystem diseases, cope with ensuing problems, and manage his/her care are remarkably diminished
Related factors: depression, apathy; fatigue
Defining characteristics: anorexia—does not eat meals when offered; states does not have an appetite, not hungry, or "I don't want to eat"; inadequate nutritional intake—eating less than body requirements; consumes minimal to none of food at most meals (i.e., consumes less than 75% of normal requirements at each or most meals); weight loss (decreased body mass from base line weight)—5% unintentional weight loss in 1 month, 10% unintentional weight loss in 6 months; physical decline (decline in bodily function)—evidence of fatigue, dehydration, incontinence of bowel and bladder; frequent exacerbation of chronic health problems such as pneumonia or urinary tract infections; cognitive decline (decline in mental processing)—as evidenced by problems with responding appropriately to environmental

stimuli, demonstrates difficulty in reasoning, decision making, judgment, memory and concentration, decreased perception; decreased social skills/social withdrawal—noticeable decrease from usual past behavior in attempts to form or participate in cooperative and interdependent relationships (e.g., decreased verbal communication with staff, family, friends); decreased participation in activities of daily living that the older person once enjoyed; self-care deficit—no longer looks after or takes charge of physical cleanliness or appearance; difficulty performing simple self-care tasks; neglects home environment; altered mood state—expresses loss of interest in pleasurable outlets such as food, sex, work, friends, family, hobbies, or entertainment; verbalizes desire for death

Family processes, altered

Definition: a change in family relationships and/or functioning

Related factors: power shift of family members; family roles shift; shift in health status of a family member; developmental transition and/or crisis; situation transition and/or crisis; informal or formal interaction with community; modification in family social status; modification in family finances

Defining characteristics: changes in power alliances; changes in assigned tasks; changes in effectiveness in completing assigned tasks; changes in mutual support; changes in availability for affective responsiveness and intimacy; changes in patterns and rituals; changes in participation in problem solving; changes in participation in decision making; changes in communication patterns; changes in availability for emotional support; changes in satisfaction with family; changes in stress-reduction behaviors; changes in expressions of conflict with and/or isolation from community resources; changes in somatic complaints; changes in expressions of conflict within family

Family processes, altered, alcoholism

Definition: the state in which the psychosocial, spiritual, and physiological functions of the family unit are chronically disorganized, leading to conflict, denial of problems, resistance to change, ineffective problem-solving, and a series of self-perpetuating crises

Related factors: abuse of alcohol; genetic predisposition; lack of problem-solving skills; inadequate coping skills; family history of alcoholism, resistance to treatment biochemical influences; addictive personality

Defining characteristics:

Roles and relationships: inconsistent parenting/low perception of parental support; ineffective spouse communication/marital problems; intimacy dysfunction; deterioration in family relationships/disturbed family dynamics; altered role function/disruption of family roles; closed communication systems; chronic family problems; family denial; lack of cohesiveness; neglected obligations; lack of skills necessary for relationships; reduced ability of family members to relate to each other for mutual growth and maturation; family unable to meet security needs of its members; disrupted family rituals; economic problems; family does not demonstrate respect for individuality and autonomy of its members; triangulating of family relationships; pattern of rejection

Behavioral: refusal to get help/inability to accept and receive help appropriately; inadequate understanding or knowledge of alcoholism; ineffective problem-solving skills; loss of control of drinking; manipulation; rationalization/denial of problems; blaming; inability to meet emotional needs of its members; alcohol abuse; broken promises; criticizing; dependency; impaired communication; difficulty with intimate relationships; enabling to maintain drinking; expression of anger inappropriately; isolation; inability to meet spiritual needs of its members; inability to express or accept wide range of feelings; inability to deal with traumatic experiences constructively; inability to adapt to change; immaturity; harsh self-judgment; lying; lack of dealing with conflict; lack of reliability; nicotine addiction; orientation toward tension relief rather than achievement of goals; seeking approval and affirmation; difficulty having fun; agitation; chaos; contradictory, paradoxical communication; diminished physical contact; disturbances in academic performance in children; disturbances in concentration; escalating conflict, failure to accomplish current or past developmental tasks; difficulty with life cycle transitions; family special occasions are alcohol centered; controlling communication/power struggles; self-blaming; stress-related physical illnesses; substance abuse other than alcohol; unresolved grief; verbal abuse of spouse or parent

Feelings: insecurity; lingering resentment; mistrust; vulnerability; rejection; repressed emotions; responsibility for alcoholic's behavior; shame/embarrassment; unhappiness; powerlessness; anger/suppressed rage; anxiety or tension or distress; emotional isolation/loneliness; frustration; guilt; hopelessness; hurt; decreased self-esteem/worthlessness; hostility; lack of identify; fear; loss; emotional control by others; misunderstood; moodiness; abandonment; being different from other people; being unloved; confused love and pity; confusion; failure; depression; dissatisfaction

Fatigue

Definition: an overwhelming sustained sense of exhaustion and decreased capacity for physical and mental work at usual level

Related factors:

Psychological: boring lifestyle; stress; anxiety; depression

Environmental: humidity; lights; noise; temperature

Situational: negative life events; occupation

Physiological: sleep deprivation; pregnancy; poor physical condition; disease states; increased physical exertion; malnutrition; anemia

Defining characteristics: inability to restore energy even after sleep; lack of energy or inability to maintain usual level of physical activity; increase in rest requirements; tired; inability to maintain usual routines; verbalization of an unremitting and overwhelming lack of energy; lethargic or listless; perceived need for additional energy to accomplish routine tasks; increase in physical complaints; compromised concentration; disinterest in surroundings, introspection; decreased performance; compromised libido; drowsy; feelings of guilt for not keeping up with responsibilities

Fear

Definition: fear is anxiety caused by consciously recognized and realistic danger. It is a perceived threat, real or imagined. Operationally, fear is the presence of immediate feeling of apprehension and fright; source known and specific; subjective responses that act as energizers but cannot be observed; and objective signs that are the result of the transformation of energy into relief behaviors and responses

Related factors: phobic stimulus or phobia; physical/social conditions; fear of others; ideas; separation from support system in potentially stressful situation; natural/innate origins; language barrier; knowledge deficit; discrepancy; environmental stimuli; learned response; sensory impairment; innate releasers; classified conditioning

Defining characteristics: dread; fight behavior-aggression; focus on "it" out there; increased alertness; panicky; flight behavior-withdrawal; worry; alarm; bed wetting; afraid; jittery; impulsiveness; ability to identify object of fear; physical arousal; concentration on the source; frightened; apprehension; immediate response to object of fear; terrified; increased heart rate; decreased self-assurance; scared; wide-eyed; attack behavior; increased tension; horror; wariness

Fluid volume, deficit

Definition: the state in which an individual experiences decreased intravascular, interstitial and/or intracellular fluid. This refers to dehydration, water loss alone without change in sodium

Related factors: active fluid volume loss; failure of regulatory mechanisms

Defining characteristics: decreased urine output; increased urine concentration; weakness; sudden weight loss (except in third-spacing); decreased venous filling; increased body temperature; decreased pulse volume/pressure; change in mental state; elevated hematocrit; decreased skin/tongue turgor; dry skin/mucous membranes; thirst; increased pulse rate; decreased blood pressure

Fluid volume deficit, risk for

Definition: the state in which an individual is at risk of experiencing vascular, cellular, or intracellular dehydration

Risk factors: factors influencing fluids needs (e.g., hypermetabolic state); medication (e.g., diuretics); loss of fluid through abnormal routes (e.g., indwelling tubes); knowledge deficiency related to fluid volume; extremes of age; deviations affecting access to or intake or absorption of fluids (e.g., physical immobility); extremes of weight; excessive losses through normal routes (e.g., diarrhea)

Fluid volume, excess

Definition: the state in which an individual experiences increased isotonic fluid retention

Related factors: compromised regulatory mechanism; excess fluid intake; excess sodium intake

Defining characteristics: jugular vein distention; decreased hemoglobin and hematocrit; weight gain over short period; dyspnea or shortness of breath; intake exceeds output; pleural effusion; orthopnea; S_3 heart sound; pulmonary artery pressure changes; oliguria; specific gravity changes; azotemia; altered electrolytes; restlessness; anxiety; anasarca; abnormal breath sounds (rales or crackles); edema; increased central venous pressure; positive hepatojugular reflex

Fluid volume imbalance, risk for

Definition: a risk of a decrease, increase, or rapid shift from one to the other of intravascular, interstitial, and/or intracellular fluid. This refers to the loss or excess or both of body fluids or replacement fluids.
Risk factors: other risk factors to be determined; scheduled for major invasive procedures

Gas exchange, impaired

Definition: excess or deficit in oxygenation and/or carbon dioxide elimination at the alveolar-capillary membrane
Related factors: ventilation perfusion imbalance; alveolar-capillary membrane changes
Defining characteristics: visual disturbances; decreased carbon dioxide; tachycardia; hypercapnia; restlessness; somnolence; irritability; hypoxia; confusion; dyspnea; abnormal arterial blood gases; cyanosis (in neonates, only); abnormal skin color (pale, dusky); hypoxemia; hypercarbia; headache upon awakening; abnormal rate, rhythm, depth of breathing; diaphoresis; abnormal arterial pH; nasal flaring

Grieving, anticipatory

Definition: intellectual and emotional responses and behaviors by which individuals, families, communities work through the process of modifying self-concept based on the perception of potential loss
Related factors: to be developed; possible non-NANDA factors: impending death; possible loss of body part or function; potential loss of significant person, possession, animal; potential loss (specify)
Defining characteristics: expressions of distress at potential loss; sorrow; guilt; denial of potential loss; anger; altered communication patterns; potential loss of significant object; denial of the significance of the loss; bargaining; alteration in eating habits, sleep patterns, dream patterns, activity level, libido; difficulty taking on new or different roles; resolution of grief prior to the reality of loss

Grieving, dysfunctional

Definition: extended, unsuccessful use of intellectual and emotional responses by which individuals, families, communities attempt to work through the process of modifying self-concept based upon the perception of loss
Related factors: actual or perceived object loss (object loss is used in the broadest sense); objects may include people, possessions, a job, status, home, ideals, parts and processes of the body
Defining characteristics: crying; sadness; reliving of past experiences with little or no reduction (diminished) of intensity of the grief; labile affect; expression of unresolved issues; interference with life functioning; verbal expression of distress at loss; idealization of lost object; difficulty in expressing loss; denial of loss; anger; alterations in: eating habits, sleep patterns, dream patterns, activity level, libido, concentration and/or pursuit of tasks; developmental regression; expression of guilt; repetitive use of ineffectual behaviors associated with attempts to reinvest in relationships; prolonged interference with life functioning; onset or exacerbation of somatic or psychosomatic responses; expression of distress at loss; reliving of past experiences

Growth, risk for altered

Definition: at risk for growth above the 97th percentile or below the 3rd percentile for age, crossing two percentile channels; disproportionate growth
Risk factors:
Prenatal: congenital/genetic disorders; maternal nutrition; multiple gestation; teratogen exposure; substance use/abuse
Individual: infection; prematurity; malnutrition; organic and inorganic factors; caregiver and/or individual maladaptive feeding behaviors; anorexia; insatiable appetite; chronic illness; substance abuse
Environmental: deprivation; teratogen exposure; lead poisoning; poverty; violence; natural disasters
Caregiver: abuse; mental illness; mental retardation; severe learning disability

Growth and development, altered

Definition: the state in which an individual demonstrates deviations in norms from his/her age group
Related factors: prescribed dependence; indifference; separation from significant others; environmental and stimulation deficiencies; effects of physical disability; inadequate care-taking; inconsistent responsiveness; multiple caretakers
Defining characteristics: altered physical growth; delay or difficulty in performing skills (motor, social, expressive) typical of age group; inability to perform self-care or self-control activities appropriate for age; flat affect; listlessness, decreased responses

Health maintenance, altered
Definition: inability to identify, manage and/or seek out help to maintain health
Related factors: ineffective individual or family coping; perceptual/cognitive impairment (complete/partial lack of gross and/or fine motor skills); lack of, or significant alteration in communication skills (written, verbal and/or gestural); unachieved developmental tasks; lack of material resources; dysfunctional grieving; disabling spiritual distress; lack of ability to make deliberate and thoughtful judgments
Defining characteristics: history of lack of health-seeking behavior; reported or observed lack of equipment, financial and/or other resources; reported or observed impairment of personal support systems; expressed interest in improving health behaviors; demonstrated lack of knowledge regarding basic health practices; demonstrated lack of adaptive behaviors to internal/external environmental changes; reported or observed inability to take responsibility for meeting basic health practices in any or all functional pattern areas

Health-seeking behaviors (specify)
Definition: a state in which an individual in stable health is actively seeking ways to alter personal health habits, and/or the environment in order to move toward a higher level of health
Related factors: to be developed
Defining characteristics: expressed or observed desire to seek a higher level of wellness; demonstrated or observed lack of knowledge in health-promotion behaviors; stated or observed unfamiliarity with wellness community resources; expression of concern about current environmental conditions on health status; expressed or observed desire for increased control of health practice

Home maintenance management, impaired
Definition: inability to independently maintain a safe growth-promoting immediate environment
Related factors: individual/family member disease or injury; unfamiliarity with neighborhood resources; lack of role modeling; lack of knowledge; insufficient family organization or planning; inadequate support systems; impaired cognitive or emotional functioning; insufficient finances
Defining characteristics:
Objective: overtaxed family members (e.g., exhausted, anxious); unwashed or unavailable cooking equipment, clothes, or linen; repeated hygienic disorders, infestations, or infections; accumulation of dirt, food wastes, or hygienic wastes; disorderly surroundings; presence of vermin or rodents; inappropriate household temperature; lack of necessary equipment or aids; offensive odors
Subjective: household members express difficulty in maintaining their home in a comfortable fashion; household members describe outstanding debts or financial crises; household requests assistance with home maintenance

Hopelessness
Definition: a subjective state in which an individual sees limited or no alternatives or personal choices available and is unable to mobilize energy on own behalf
Related factors: abandonment; prolonged activity restriction creating isolation; lost belief in transcendent values/God; long-term stress; failing or deteriorating physical condition
Defining characteristics: passivity; decreased verbalization; verbal cues (e.g., despondent content, "I can't," sighing); closing eyes; decreased affect; decreased appetite; decreased response to stimuli; increased/decreased sleep; lack of initiative; lack of involvement in care/passively allowing care; shrugging in response to speaker; turning away from speaker

Hyperthermia
Definition: a state in which an individual's body temperature is elevated above normal range
Related factors: illness or trauma; increased metabolic rate; vigorous activity; medications or anesthesia; inability or decreased ability to perspire; [prolonged] exposure to hot environment; dehydration; inappropriate clothing
Defining characteristics: increase in body temperature above normal range; seizures or convulsions; flushed skin; increased respiratory rate; tachycardia; [skin] warm to touch

Hypothermia
Definition: the state in which an individual's body temperature is reduced below normal range

Related factors: exposure to cool or cold environment; medications causing vasodilation; malnutrition; inadequate clothing; illness or trauma; evaporation from skin in cool environment; decreased metabolic rate; damage to hypothalamus; consumption of alcohol; aging; inability or decreased ability to shiver; inactivity

Defining characteristics: pallor; reduction in body temperature below normal range; shivering; cool skin; cyanotic nail beds; hypertension; piloerection; slow capillary refill; tachycardia

Incontinence, bowel

Definition: change in normal bowel habits characterized by involuntary passage of stool

Related factors: environmental factors (e.g., inaccessible bathroom); incomplete emptying of bowel; rectal sphincter abnormality; impaction; dietary habits; colorectal lesions; stress; lower motor nerve damage; abnormally high abdominal or intestinal pressure; general decline in muscle tone; loss of rectal sphincter control; impaired cognition; upper motor nerve damage; chronic diarrhea; self-care deficit-toileting; impaired reservoir capacity; medications; immobility; laxative abuse

Defining characteristics: constant dribbling of soft stool; fecal odor; inability to delay defecation; urgency; self-report of inability to feel rectal fullness; fecal staining of clothing and/or bedding; recognizes rectal fullness but reports inability to expel formed stool; inattention to urge to defecate; inability to recognize urge to defecate; red perianal skin

Incontinence, functional urinary

Definition: inability of usually continent person to reach toilet in time to avoid unintentional loss of urine

Related factors: psychological factors; impaired vision; impaired cognition; neuromuscular limitations; altered environmental factors; weakened supporting pelvic structures

Defining characteristics: may only be incontinent in early morning; senses need to void; amount of time required to reach toilet exceeds length of time between sensing urge and uncontrolled voiding; loss of urine before reaching toilet; able to completely empty bladder

Incontinence, reflex urinary

Definition: an involuntary loss of urine at somewhat predictable intervals when a specific bladder volume is reached

Related factors: tissue damage from radiation cystitis, inflammatory bladder conditions, or radical pelvic surgery; neurological impairment above level of sacral micturition center or pontine micturition center

Defining characteristics: no sensation of urge to void; complete emptying with lesion above pontine micturition center; incomplete emptying with lesion above sacral micturition center; no sensation of bladder fullness; sensations associated with full bladder such as sweating, restlessness, and abdominal discomfort; unable to cognitively inhibit or initiate voiding; no sensation of voiding; predictable pattern of voiding; sensation to urinate without voluntary inhibition of bladder contraction.

Incontinence, stress urinary

Definition: the state in which an individual experiences a loss of urine of less than 50 ml occurring with increased abdominal pressure

Related factors: weak pelvic muscles and structural supports; over distention between voidings; incompetent bladder outlet; degenerative changes in pelvic muscles and structural supports associated with increased age; high intra-abdominal pressure (e.g., obesity, gravid uterus)

Defining characteristics: reported or observed dribbling with increased abdominal pressure; urinary frequency (more often than every 2 hours); urinary urgency

Incontinence, total urinary

Definition: the state in which an individual experiences a continuous and unpredictable loss of urine

Related factors: neuropathy preventing transmission of reflex indicating bladder fullness; trauma or disease affecting spinal cord nerves; anatomic (fistula); independent contraction of detrusor reflex due to surgery; neurological dysfunction causing triggering of micturition at unpredictable times

Defining characteristics: constant flow of urine occurs at unpredictable times without distention or uninhibited bladder contractions/spasm; nocturia; unsuccessful incontinence refractory treatments; unawareness of incontinence; lack of perineal or bladder filling awareness

Incontinence, urge urinary

Definition: the state in which an individual experiences involuntary passage of urine occurring soon after a strong sense of urgency to void

Related factors: alcohol; caffeine; decreased bladder capacity (e.g., history of PID, abdominal surgeries, indwelling (urinary catheter); increased fluid intake; increased urine concentration; irritation of bladder stretch receptors causing spasm (e.g., bladder infection); over distention of bladder

Defining characteristics: urinary urgency; bladder contracture/spasm; frequency (voiding more often than every two hours); voiding in large amounts (more than 550 cc); voiding in small amounts (less than 100 cc); nocturia (more than two times a night); inability to reach toilet in time

Infant behavior, disorganized

Definition: disintegrated physiological and neurobehavioral responses to the environment

Related factors:

Prenatal: congenital or genetic disorders; teratogenic exposure

Postnatal: malnutrition; oral/motor problems; pain; feeding intolerance; invasive/painful procedures; prematurity

Individual: illness; immature neurological system; gestational age; postconceptual age

Environmental: physical environment inappropriateness; sensory inappropriateness; sensory overstimulation; sensory deprivation

Caregiver: cue misreading; cue knowledge deficit; environmental stimulation contribution

Defining characteristics:

Regulatory problems: inability to inhibit (inability to look away from stimulus); irritability

State-organization system: active-awake (fussy, worried gaze); diffuse/unclear sleep; state oscillation; quiet-awake (staring, gaze aversion); irritable or panicky crying

Attention-interaction system: abnormal response to sensory stimuli (e.g., difficult to soothe, inability to sustain alert status)

Motor system: increased, decreased, or limp tone; finger splay, fisting or hands to face; hyperextension of arms and legs; tremors, startles, twitches, jittery, jerky, uncoordinated movement; altered primitive reflexes

Physiological: bradycardia, tachycardia, or arrhythmias; pale, cyanotic, mottled, or flushed color; bradypnea, tachypnea, apnea; "time-out signals" (e.g., gaze, grasp, hiccup, cough, sneeze, sigh, slack jaw, open mouth, tongue thrust); oximeter desaturation; feeding intolerance (aspiration or emesis)

Infant behavior, risk for disorganized

Definition: risk for alteration in integrating and modulation of physiological and behavioral systems of functioning (i.e., autonomic, motor, state, organizational, self-regulatory, and attentional-interactional systems)

Risk factors: invasive/painful procedures; lack of containment/boundaries; oral/motor problems; pain; prematurity; environmental overstimulation

Infant behavior, organized, potential for enhanced

Definition: a pattern of modulation of the physiologic and behavioral systems of functioning (i.e., autonomic, motor, state organizational, self-regulators, and attentional-interactional systems) in an infant that is satisfactory but that can be improved, resulting in higher levels of integration in response to environmental stimuli

Related factors: pain; prematurity

Defining characteristics: definite sleep-wake states; use of some self-regulatory behaviors; response to visual/auditory stimuli; stable physiologic measures

Infant feeding pattern, ineffective

Definition: a state in which an infant demonstrates an impaired ability to suck or coordinate the suck-swallow response

Related factors: prolonged NPO; anatomic abnormality; neurological impairment/delay; oral hypersensitivity; prematurity

Defining characteristics: inability to coordinate sucking, swallowing and breathing; inability to initiate or sustain an effective suck

Infection, risk for
Definition: the state in which an individual is at increased risk for being invaded by pathogenic organisms
Risk factors: invasive procedures; insufficient knowledge to avoid exposure to pathogens; trauma; tissue destruction and increased environmental exposure; rupture of amniotic membranes; pharmaceutical agents; malnutrition; increased environmental exposure; immunosuppression; inadequate acquired immunity; inadequate secondary defenses (decreased hemoglobin, leukopenia, suppressed inflammatory response); inadequate primary defenses (broken skin, traumatized tissue, decrease in ciliary action, stasis of body fluids, change in pH secretions, altered peristalsis); chronic disease.

Injury, risk for
Definition: a state in which an individual is at risk of injury as a result of environmental conditions interacting with the individual's adaptive and defensive resources
Risk factors:
External: mode of transport or transportation; people or provider (e.g., nosocomial agents, staffing patterns, cognitive, affective and psychomotor factors); physical (e.g., design, structure, and arrangement of community, building and/or equipment); nutrients (e.g., vitamins, food types); biological (e.g., immunization level of community, microorganism); chemical (e.g., pollutants, poisons, drugs, pharmaceutical agents, alcohol, caffeine, nicotine, preservatives, cosmetics, and dyes)
Internal: psychological (affective orientation); malnutrition; abnormal blood profile (e.g., leukocytosis/leukopenia); altered clotting factors; thrombocytopenia; sickle cell; thalassemia; decreased hemoglobin; immune-autoimmune dysfunction; biochemical, regulatory function (e.g., sensory dysfunction); integrative dysfunction; effector dysfunction; tissue hypoxia; developmental age (physiological, psychosocial); physical (e.g., broken skin, altered mobility)

Knowledge deficit (specify)
Definition: absence or deficiency of cognitive information related to a specific topic
Related factors: cognitive limitation; information misinterpretation; lack of exposure; lack of interest in learning; lack of recall; unfamiliarity with information resources
Defining characteristics: verbalization of the problem; inappropriate or exaggerated behaviors (e.g., hysterical, hostile, agitated, apathetic); inaccurate follow-through of instruction; inaccurate performance of test

Latex allergy response
Definition: an allergic response to natural latex rubber products
Related factors: no immune mechanism response
Defining characteristics:
Type I reactions: immediate
Type IV reactions: eczema; irritation; reaction to additives causes discomfort (e.g., thiurams, carbamates); redness; delayed onset (hours)
Irritant reactions: erythema; chapped or cracked skin; blisters

Latex allergy response, risk for
Definition: at risk for allergic response to natural latex rubber products
Risk factors: multiple surgical procedures, especially from infancy (e.g., spina bifida); allergies to bananas, avocados, tropical fruits, kiwi, chestnuts; professions with daily exposure to latex (e.g., medicine, nursing, dentistry); conditions needing continuous or intermittent catheterization; history of reactions to latex (e.g., balloons, condoms, gloves); allergies to poinsettia plants; history of allergies and asthma

Loneliness, risk for
Definition: a subjective state in which an individual is at risk of experiencing vague dysphoria
Risk factors: affectional deprivation; social isolation; cathetic deprivation; physical isolation

Management of therapeutic regimen: community, ineffective
Definition: a pattern of regulating and integrating into community processes programs for treatment of illness and the sequelae of illness that are unsatisfactory for meeting health-related goals
Related factors: to be developed

Defining characteristics: illness symptoms above the norm expected for the number and type of population; unexpected acceleration of illness(es); number of health care resources are insufficient for the incidence or prevalence of illness (es); deficits in people and programs to be accountable for illness care of aggregates; deficits in community activities for secondary and tertiary prevention; deficits in advocates for aggregates; unavailable health care resources for illness care

Management of therapeutic regimen: families, ineffective
Definition: a pattern of regulating and integrating into family processes a program for treatment of illness and the sequelae of illness that is unsatisfactory for meeting specific health goals
Related factors: complexity of health care system; complexity of therapeutic regime; decisional conflicts; economic difficulties; excessive demands made on individual or family; family conflict
Defining characteristics: inappropriate family activities for meeting the goals of a treatment or prevention program; acceleration of illness symptoms of a family member; lack of attention to illness and its sequelae; verbalized difficulty with regulation/integration of one or more effects or prevention of complications; verbalized desire to manage the treatment of illness and prevention of the sequelae; verbalizes that family did not take action to reduce risk factors for progression of illness and sequelae

Management of therapeutic regimen: individual, effective
Definition: a pattern of regulating and integrating into daily living a program for treatment of illness and its sequelae that is satisfactory for meeting specific health goals
Related factors: to be developed; [wellness nursing diagnosis]
Defining characteristics: appropriate choices of daily activities for meeting the goals of a treatment or prevention program; illness symptoms are within a normal range of expectation; verbalized desire to manage the treatment of illness and prevention of sequelae; verbalized intent to reduce risk factors for progression of illness and sequelae

Management of therapeutic regimen: individuals, ineffective
Definition: a pattern of regulating and integrating into daily living a program for treatment of illness and the sequelae of illness that is unsatisfactory for meeting specific health goals
Related factors: perceived barriers; social support deficits; powerlessness; perceived susceptibility; perceived benefits; mistrust of regimen and/or health care personnel; knowledge deficits; family patterns of health care; family conflict; excessive demands made on individual or family; economic difficulties; decisional conflicts; complexity of therapeutic regime; complexity of health care system; perceived seriousness; inadequate number and types of cues to action
Defining characteristics: choices of daily living ineffective for meeting the goals of a treatment or prevention program; verbalized desire to manage the treatment of illness and prevention of sequelae; verbalized that did not take action to reduce risk factors for progression of illness and sequelae; verbalized difficulty with regulation/integration of one or more prescribed regimens for treatment of illness and its effects or prevention of complications; acceleration of illness symptoms; verbalized that did not take action to include treatment regimens in daily routines

Memory, impaired
Definition: the state in which an individual experiences the inability to remember or recall bits of information or behavioral skills. Impaired memory may be attributed to pathophysiological or situational causes that are either temporary or permanent
Related factors: fluid and electrolyte imbalance; neurological disturbances; excessive environmental disturbances; anemia; acute or chronic hypoxia; decreased cardiac output
Defining characteristics: inability to recall factual information; inability to recall recent or past events; inability to learn or retain new skills or information; inability to determine if a behavior was performed; observed or reported experiences of forgetting; inability to perform a previously learned skill; forgets to perform a behavior at a scheduled time

Mobility, impaired bed
Definition: limitation of independent movement from one bed position to another [specify level]
Suggested Functional Level Classification:
0 = is completely independent
1 = requires use of equipment or device

2 = requires help from another person for assistance, supervision, or teaching
3 = requires help from another person and equipment/device
4 = is dependent; does not participate in activity
Related factors: to be developed
Defining characteristics: impaired ability to turn side to side; impaired ability to move from supine to sitting or sitting to supine; impaired ability to "scoot" or reposition self in bed; impaired ability to move from supine to prone or prone to supine; impaired ability to move from supine to long sitting or long sitting to supine

Mobility, impaired physical
Definition: a limitation in independent, purposeful physical movement of the body or of one or more extremities [specify level]
Suggested Functional Level Classification:
0 = is completely independent
1 = requires use of equipment or device
2 = requires help from another person, for assistance, supervision, or teaching
3 = requires help from another person and equipment/device
4 = is dependent; does not participate in activity
Related factors: medications; prescribed movement restrictions; discomfort; lack of knowledge regarding value of physical activity; body mass index above 75th age-appropriate percentile; sensoriperceptual impairments; neuromuscular impairment; pain; musculoskeletal impairment; intolerance to activity/decreased strength and endurance; depressive mood state or anxiety; cognitive impairment; decreased muscle strength, control and/or mass; reluctance to initiate movement; sedentary lifestyle or disuse or deconditioning; selective or generalized malnutrition; loss of integrity of bone structures; developmental delay; joint stiffness or contractures; limited cardiovascular endurance; altered cellular metabolism; lack of physical or social environmental supports; cultural beliefs regarding age appropriate activity
Defining characteristics: postural instability during performance of routine activities of daily living; limited ability to perform gross motor skills; limited ability to perform fine motor skills; uncoordinated or jerky movements; limited range of motion; difficulty turning; decreased reaction time; movement-induced shortness of breath; gait changes (e.g., decreased walk, speed, difficulty initiating gait, small steps, shuffles feet, exaggerated lateral postural sway); engages in substitutions for movement (e.g., increased attention to other's activity, controlling behavior, focus on pre-illness/disability activity); slowed movement; movement-induced tremor

Mobility, impaired wheelchair
Definition: limitation of independent operation of wheelchair within environment [specify level]
Suggested Functional Level Classification:
0 = is completely independent
1 = requires use of equipment or device
2 = requires help from another person for assistance, supervision, or teaching
3 = requires help from another person and equipment/device
4 = is dependent; does not participate in activity
Related factors: to be developed
Defining characteristics: impaired ability to operate manual or power wheelchair on even or uneven surface; impaired ability to operate manual or power wheelchair on an incline or decline; impaired ability to operate wheelchair on curbs

Nausea
Definition: an unpleasant, wave-like sensation in the back of the throat, epigastrium, or throughout the abdomen that may or may not lead to vomiting
Related factors: chemotherapy; post-surgical anesthesia; irritation to the gastrointestinal system; stimulation of neuropharmacologic mechanisms
Defining characteristics: usually precedes vomiting, but may be experienced after vomiting or when vomiting does not occur; accompanied by pallor, cold and clammy skin, increased salivation, tachycardia, gastric stasis, and diarrhea; accompanied by swallowing movements affected by skeletal muscles; reports "nausea" or "sick to stomach"

Noncompliance (specify)
Definition: the extent to which a person's and/or caregiver's behavior coincides or fails to coincide with a health-promoting or therapeutic plan agreed upon by the person (and/or family, and/or community) and health care professional. In the presence of an agreed-upon, health-promoting or therapeutic plan, person's or caregiver's behavior may be fully, partially, or nonadherent and may lead to clinically effective, partially effective, on ineffective outcomes.
Related factors:
Health care plan: duration; significant others; cost; intensity; complexity
Individual factors: personal and developmental abilities; health beliefs; cultural influences; spiritual values; individual's value system; knowledge and skill relevant to the regime behavior; motivational forces
Health system: satisfaction with care; credibility of provider; access and convenience of care; financial flexibility of plan; client-provider relationships; provider reimbursement of teaching and follow-up; provider continuity and regular follow-up; individual health coverage; communication and teaching skills of the provider
Network: involvement of members in health plan; social value regarding plan; perceived beliefs of significant others
Defining characteristics: behavior indicative of failure to adhere (by direct observation or by statements of patient or significant others); evidence of development of complications; evidence of exacerbation of symptoms; failure to keep appointments; failure to progress; objective tests (e.g., physiological measures, detection of physiologic markers)

Nutrition, altered: less than body requirements
Definition: the state in which an individual is experiencing an intake of nutrients insufficient to meet metabolic needs
Related factors: inability to ingest or digest food or absorb nutrients due to biological, psychological, or economic factors
Defining characteristics: pale conjunctival and mucous membranes; weakness of muscles required for swallowing or mastication; sore, inflamed buccal cavity; satiety immediately after ingesting food; reported or evidence of lack of food; reported inadequate food intake less than RDA (recommended daily allowance); reported altered taste sensation; perceived inability to ingest food; misconceptions; loss of weight with adequate food intake; aversion to eating; abdominal cramping; poor muscle tone; abdominal pain with or without pathology; lack of interest in food; body weight 20% or more under ideal; capillary fragility; diarrhea and/or steatorrhea; excessive loss of hair; hyperactive bowel sounds; lack of information, misinformation

Nutrition, altered: more than body requirements
Definition: the state in which an individual is experiencing an intake of nutrients that exceeds metabolic needs
Related factors: excessive intake in relation to metabolic need
Defining characteristics: triceps skin fold greater than 25 mm in women; weight 20% over ideal for height and frame; triceps skin fold greater than 15 mm in men; eating in response to external cues, such as time of day, social situation; eating in response to internal cues other than hunger (e.g., anxiety); reported or observed dysfunctional eating pattern pairing food with other activities; sedentary activity level; concentrating food intake at the end of the day

Nutrition, altered: risk for more than body requirements
Definition: the state in which an individual is at risk of experiencing an intake of nutrients that exceeds metabolic needs
Risk factors: reported use of solid food as major food source before 5 months of age; concentrating food intake at end of day; reported or observed obesity in one or both parents; reported or observed higher baseline weight at beginning of each pregnancy; rapid transition across growth percentiles in infants or children; pairing food with other activities; observed use of food as reward or comfort measure; eating in response to internal cues other than hunger such as anxiety; eating in response to external cues such as time of day, social situation; dysfunctional eating patterns

Oral mucous membrane, altered
Definition: disruptions of the lips and soft tissue of the oral cavity
Related factors: chemotherapy; chemical (e.g., alcohol, tobacco, acidic foods, regular use of inhalers); depression; immunosuppression; aging-related loss of connective, adipose, or bone tissue; barriers to professional care; cleft lip or palate; medication side effects; lack of or decreased salivation; trauma (chemical, e.g., acidic foods, drugs, noxious agents, alcohol); pathological conditions - oral cavity (radiation to head or neck); NPO for more than 24 hours; mouth breathing; malnutrition or vitamin deficiency; dehydration; infection; ineffective oral hygiene; mechanical (e.g., ill-

fitting dentures, braces, tubes [endotracheal/nasogastric], surgery in oral cavity); decreased platelets; immunocompromised; impaired salivation; radiation therapy; barriers to oral self-care; diminished hormone levels (women); stress; loss of supportive structures

Defining characteristics: purulent drainage or exudates; gingival recession, pockets deeper than 4 mm; enlarged tonsils beyond what is developmentally appropriate; smooth atrophic, sensitive tongue; geographic tongue; mucosal dendation; presence of pathogens; difficult speech; self-report of bad taste; gingival or mucosal pallor; oral pain/discomfort; xerostomia (dry mouth); vesicles, nodules, or papules; white patches/plaques, spongy patches or white curd-like exudate; oral lesions or ulcers; halitosis; edema; hyperemia; desquamation; coated tongue; stomatitis; self-report of difficulty eating or swallowing; self-report of diminished or absent taste; bleeding; macroplasia; gingival hyperplasia; fissures, chelitis; red or bluish masses (e.g., hemangiomas)

Pain

Definition: an unpleasant sensory and emotional experience arising from actual or potential tissue damage or described in terms of such damage (International Association for the Study of Pain); sudden or slow onset of any intensity from mild to severe and a duration of less than 6 months

Related factors: injuring agents (biological, chemical, physical, psychological)

Defining characteristics: verbal or coded report; observed evidence [of pain]; antalgic position; protective behavior; guarding behavior; antalgic gestures; facial mask; sleep disturbance (eyes lackluster, "hecohe [beaten] look," fixed or scattered movement, grimace); self-focus; narrowed focus (altered time perception, impaired thought processes, reduced interaction with people and environment); distraction behavior (e.g., pacing, seeking out other people and/or activities, repetitive activities); autonomic responses (e.g., diaphoresis, blood pressure, respiration, pulse change, pupillary dilation); autonomic alteration in muscle tone (may span from listless to rigid); expressive behavior (e.g., restlessness, moaning, crying, vigilance, irritability, sighing); changes in appetite and eating

Pain, chronic

Definition: an unpleasant sensory and emotional experience arising from actual or potential tissue damage or described in terms of such damage (International Association for the Study of Pain); sudden or slow onset of any intensity from mild to severe, constant or recurring without an anticipated or predictable end and a duration of greater than 6 months

Related factors: chronic physical/psychosocial disability (e.g., cancer, arthritis)

Defining characteristics: weight changes; verbal or coded report or observed evidence of protective behavior; verbal or coded report or observed evidence of guarding behavior; verbal or coded report or observed evidence of facial mask; verbal or coded report or observed evidence of irritability; verbal or coded report or observed evidence of self-focusing; verbal or coded report or observed evidence of restlessness; verbal or coded report or observed evidence of depression; atrophy of involved muscle group; changes in sleep pattern; fatigue; fear of reinjury; reduced interaction with people; altered ability to continue previous activities; sympathetic mediated responses (e.g., temperature, cold, changes of body position, hypersensitivity); anorexia

Parent/infant/child attachment, risk for altered

Definition: disruption of the interactive process between parent/significant other and infant that fosters the development of a protective and nurturing reciprocal relationship

Risk factors: physical barriers; anxiety associated with the parent role; substance abuse; premature infant; ill infant/child who is unable to effectively initiate parental contact due to altered behavioral organization; lack of privacy; inability of parents to meet the personal needs; separation

Parental role conflict

Definition: the state in which a parent experiences role confusion and conflict in response to crisis

Related factors: change in marital status; home care of a child with special needs (e.g., apnea monitoring, postural drainage, hyperalimentation); interruptions of family life due to home care regimen (e.g., treatments, caregivers, lack of respite); specialized care centers, policies; separation from child due to chronic illness; intimidation with invasive or restrictive modalities (e.g., isolation, intubation)

Defining characteristics: parent(s) express concern(s) about changes in parental role, family functioning, family communication, family health; parent(s) expresses concern(s)/feeling(s) of inadequacy to provide for child/s physical and emotional needs during hospitalization or in home; demonstrated disruption in care taking routines; expresses concern about perceived loss of control over decisions relating to their child; reluctant to participate in usual care-taking activities even with encouragement and support; verbalizes or demonstrates feelings of guilt, anger, fear, anxiety and/or frustrations about effect of child's illness on family process

Parenting, altered

Definition: inability of the primary caretaker to create an environment that promotes the optimum growth and development of the child

Related factors:

Social: Lack of access to resources; social isolation; lack of resources; poor home environments; lack of family cohesiveness; inadequate child care arrangements; lack of transportation; unemployment or job problems; role strain or overload; marital conflict, declining satisfaction; lack of value of parenthood; change in family unit; low socioeconomic class; unplanned or unwanted pregnancy; presence of stress (e.g., financial, legal, recent crisis, cultural move); lack of, or poor, parental role model; single parents; lack of social support networks; father or child not involved; history of being abusive; history of being abused; financial difficulties; maladaptive coping strategies; poverty; poor problem-solving skills; inability to put child's needs before own; low self-esteem; relocations; legal difficulties

Knowledge: lack of knowledge about child health maintenance; lack of knowledge about parenting skills; unrealistic expectation for self, infant, partner; limited cognitive functioning; lack of knowledge about child development; inability to recognize and act on infant cues; low educational level or attainment; poor communication skills; lack of cognitive readiness for parenthood; preference for physical punishment

Physiological: physical illness

Infant or child: premature birth; illness; prolonged separation from parent; not gender desired; attention deficit hyperactivity disorder; difficult temperament; separation from parent at birth; lack of goodness of fit (temperament) with parental expectations; unplanned or unwanted child; handicapping condition or developmental delay; multiple births; altered perceptual abilities

Psychological: history of substance abuse or dependencies; disability; depression; difficult labor and/or delivery; young age, especially adolescent; history of mental illness; high number of closely spaced pregnancies; sleep deprivation or disruption; lack of, or late, prenatal care; separation from infant/child; multiple births

Defining characteristics:

Infant or child: poor academic performance; frequent illness; runaway; incidence of physical and psychological trauma or abuse; frequent accidents; lack of attachment; failure to thrive; behavioral disorders; poor social competence; lack of separation anxiety; poor cognitive development

Parental: inappropriate child care arrangements; rejection or hostility to child; statement of inability to meet child's needs; inflexibility to meet needs of child, situation; poor or inappropriate catering skills; high punitiveness; inconsistent care; child abuse; inadequate child health maintenance; unsafe home environment; verbalization, cannot control child; negative statements about child; verbalization of role inadequacy frustration; inappropriate visual, tactile, auditory stimulation; inappropriate child care arrangements; abandonment; insecure or lack of attachment to infant; inconsistent behavior management; child neglect; little cuddling; maternal-child interaction deficit; poor parent-child interaction

Parenting, altered, risk for

Definition: risk for inability of the primary caretaker to create, maintain, or regain an environment that promotes the optimum growth and development of the child

Risk factors:

Social: marital conflict, declining satisfaction; history of being abused; poor problem solving skills; role strain/overload; social isolation; legal difficulties; lack of access to resources; lack of value of parenthood; relocation; poverty; poor home environment; lack of family cohesiveness; lack of poor parental role model; father of child not involved; history of being abused; financial difficulties; low self-esteem; unplanned or unwanted pregnancy; inadequate child care arrangements; maladaptive coping strategies; lack of resources; low socioeconomic class; lack of transportation; change in family unit; unemployment or job problems; single parent; lack of social support network; inability to put child's needs before own; stress

Knowledge: low educational level or attainment; unrealistic expectations of child; lack of knowledge about parenting skills; poor communication skills; preference for physical punishment; inability to recognize and act on infant cues; low

cognitive functioning; lack of knowledge about child health maintenance; lack of knowledge about child development; lack of cognitive readiness for parenthood
Physiological: physical illness
Infant or child: multiple births; handicapping condition or developmental delay; illness; altered perceptual abilities; lack of goodness of fit (temperament) with parental expectations; unplanned or unwanted child; premature birth; not gender desired; difficult temperament; attention deficit hyperactivity disorder; prolonged separation from parent; separation from parent at birth
Psychological: separation from infant/child; high number of closely spaced children; disability; sleep deprivation or disruption; multiple births; difficult labor and/or delivery; young ages, especially adolescent; depression; history of mental illness; lack of, or late, prenatal care; history of substance abuse or dependence

Perioperative positioning injury, risk for
Definition: a state in which the client is at risk for injury as a result of the environmental conditions found in the perioperative setting
Risk factors: disorientation; edema; emaciation; immobilization, muscle weakness; obesity; sensory/perceptual disturbances due to anesthesia

Peripheral neurovascular dysfunction, risk for
Definition: a state in which an individual is at risk of experiencing a disruption in circulation, sensation or motion of an extremity
Risk factors: trauma; vascular obstruction; orthopedic surgery; fractures; burns; mechanical compression (e.g., tourniquet, cast, brace, dressing or restraint); immobilization

Personal identify disturbance
Definition: inability to distinguish between self and nonself
Related factors: to be developed
Defining characteristics: to be developed

Poisoning, risk for
Definition: accentuated risk of accidental exposure to or ingestion of drugs or dangerous products in doses sufficient to cause poisoning
Risk factors:
External: unprotected contact with heavy metals or chemicals; medicines stored in unlocked cabinets accessible to children or confused people; presence of poisonous vegetation; presence of atmospheric pollutants; paint, lacquer, etc., in poorly ventilated areas or without effective protection; flaking, peeling paint or plaster in presence of young children; chemical contamination of food and water; availability of illicit drugs potentially contaminated by poisonous additives; large supplies of drugs in house; dangerous products placed or stored within reach of children or confused people
Internal: verbalization of occupational setting without adequate safeguards; reduced vision; lack of safety or drug education; lack of proper precaution; insufficient finances; cognitive or emotional difficulties

Post-trauma syndrome
Definition: a sustained maladaptive response to a traumatic, overwhelming event
Related factors: events outside the range of usual human experience; physical and psychosocial abuse; tragic occurrence involving multiple deaths; sudden destruction of one's home or community; epidemics; being held prisoner of war or criminal victimization (torture); wars; rape; natural disasters and/or man-made disasters; serious accidents; witnessing mutilation, violent death, or other horrors; serious threat or injury to self or loved ones; industrial and motor vehicle accidents; military combat
Defining characteristics: avoidance; repression; difficulty in concentrating; grief; intrusive thoughts; neurosensory irritability; palpitations; enuresis (in children); anger and/or rage; intrusive dreams; nightmares; aggression; hypervigilant; exaggerated startle response; hopelessness; altered mood states; shame; panic attacks; alienation; denial; horror; substance abuse; depression; anxiety; guilt; fear; gastric irritability; detachment; psychogenic amnesia; irritability; numbing; compulsive behavior; flashbacks; headaches

Post-trauma syndrome, risk for

Definition: a risk for sustained maladaptive response to a traumatic, overwhelming event

Risk factors: occupation (e.g., police, fire, rescue, corrections, emergency room staff, mental health); exaggerated sense of responsibility; perception of event; survivor's role in the event; displacement from home; inadequate social support; non-supportive environment; diminished ego strength; duration of the event

Powerlessness

Definition: perception that one's own action will not significantly affect an outcome; a perceived lack of control over a current situation or immediate happening

Related factors: health care environment; illness-related regime; interpersonal interaction; lifestyle of helplessness

Defining characteristics:

Low: expressions of uncertainty about fluctuating energy levels; passivity

Moderate: nonparticipation in care or decision making when opportunities are provided; resentment; anger; guilt; reluctance to express true feelings; passivity; dependence on others that may result in irritability; fearing alienation from caregivers; expressions of dissatisfaction and frustration over inability to perform previous tasks and/or activities; expression of doubt regarding role performance; does not monitor progress; does not defend self-care practices when challenged; inability to seek information regarding care

Severe: verbal expressions of having no control or influence over self-care, situation, or outcome; apathy; depression over physical deterioration that occurs despite patient compliance with regimens

Protection, altered

Definition: the state in which an individual experiences a decrease in the ability to guard self from internal or external threat such as illness or injury

Related factors: abnormal blood profiles (e.g., leukopenia, thrombocytopenia, anemia, coagulation); inadequate nutrition; extremes of age; drug therapies (e.g., antineoplastic, corticosteroid, immune, anticoagulant, thrombolytic); alcohol abuse; treatments (e.g., surgery, radiation); diseases such as cancer and immune disorders

Defining characteristics: maladaptive stress response; neuro-sensory alteration; impaired healing; deficient immunity; altered clotting; dyspnea; insomnia; weakness; restlessness; pressure ulcers; perspiring; itching; immobility; fatigue; anorexia

Rape-trauma syndrome

Definition: sustained maladaptive response to a forced, violent sexual penetration against the victim's will and consent

Related factors: rape

Defining characteristics: disorganization; change in relationships; confusion; physical trauma (e.g., bruising, tissue irritation); suicide attempts; denial; guilt; paranoia; humiliation; embarrassment; aggression; muscle tension and/or spasms; mood swings; dependence; powerlessness; nightmares and sleep disturbances; sexual dysfunction; revenge; phobias; loss of self-esteem; inability to make decisions; dissociative disorders; self-blame; hyperalertness; vulnerability; substance abuse; depression; helplessness; anger; anxiety; agitation; shame; shock; fear

Rape-trauma syndrome: compound reaction

Definition: forced violent sexual penetration against the victim's will and consent. The trauma syndrome that develops from this attack or attempted attack includes an acute phase of disorganization of the victim's lifestyle and a long-term process of reorganization of lifestyle.

Related factors: to be developed

Defining characteristics: change in lifestyle (e.g., changes in residence, dealing with repetitive nightmares and phobias, seeking family support, needing social network support in long-term phase); emotional reaction (e.g., anger, embarrassment, fear of physical violence and death, humiliation, revenge, self-blame in acute phase); multiple physical symptoms (e.g., gastrointestinal irritability, genitourinary discomfort, muscle tension, sleep pattern disturbance in acute phase); reactivated symptoms of such previous conditions (i.e., physical illness, psychiatric illness in acute phase); reliance on alcohol and/or drugs (acute phase)

Rape-trauma syndrome: silent reaction

Definition: forced violent sexual penetration against the victim's will and consent. The trauma syndrome that develops from this attack or attempted attack includes an acute phase of disorganization of the victim's lifestyle and a long-term process or reorganization of lifestyle.

Related factors: to be developed

Defining characteristics: increased anxiety during interview (i.e., blocking of associations, long periods of silence, minor stuttering, physical distress); sudden onset of phobic reaction; no verbalization of the occurrence of rape; abrupt changes in relationships with men; increase in nightmares; pronounced changes in sexual behavior

Relocation stress syndrome

Definition: physiological and/or psychosocial disturbances as a result of transfer from one environment to another

Related factors: impaired psychosocial health status; past, concurrent, and recent losses; moderate to high degree of environment change; losses involved with decision to move; lack of adequate support system; history and types of previous transfers; feeling of powerlessness; decreased physical health status; little or no preparation for the impending move

Defining characteristics: increased confusion; loneliness; depression; apprehension; anxiety; change in environment/location; sleep disturbance; withdrawal; weight change; vigilance; verbalization of unwillingness to relocate; verbalization of being concerned/upset about transfer; sad affect; restlessness; lack of trust; insecurity; increased verbalization of needs; gastrointestinal disturbances; dependency; change in eating habits; unfavorable comparison of post/pre-transfer staff

Role performance, altered

Definition: the patterns of behavior and self-expression do not match the environmental context, norms, and expectations

Related factors:

Social: inadequate or inappropriate linkage with the health care system; job schedule demands; young age, developmental level; lack of rewards; poverty; family conflict; inadequate support system; inadequate role socialization (e.g., role model, expectations, responsibilities); low social economic status; stress and conflict; domestic violence; lack of resources

Knowledge: inadequate role preparation (e.g., role transition, skill, rehearsal, validation); lack of knowledge about role; role transition; lack of opportunity for role rehearsal; developmental transitions; unrealistic role expectations; education attainment level; lack of or inadequate role model; lack of knowledge about role skills

Physiological: inadequate/inappropriate linkage with health care system; substance abuse; mental illness; body image alteration; physical illness; cognitive deficits; health alterations (e.g., physical health, body image, self-esteem, mental health, psychosocial health, cognition, learning style, neurological health); depression; low self-esteem; pain; fatigue

Defining characteristics: change in self-perception of role; role denial; inadequate external support for role enactment; inadequate adaptation to change or transition; system conflict; change in usual patterns of responsibility; discrimination; domestic violence; harassment; uncertainty; altered role perceptions; role strain; inadequate self-management; role ambivalence; pessimistic; inadequate motivation; inadequate confidence; inadequate role competency and skills; inadequate knowledge; inappropriate developmental expectations; role conflict; role confusion; powerlessness; inadequate coping; anxiety or depression; role overload; change in other's perception of role; change in capacity to resume role; role dissatisfaction; inadequate opportunities for role enactment

Self-care deficit, bathing/hygiene

Definition: impaired ability to perform or complete bathing/hygiene activities for oneself (see functional level classification under diagnosis *Impaired Physical Mobility*)

Risk factors: discomfort

Related factors: decreased or lack of motivation; weakness and tiredness; severe anxiety; inadequate to perceive body part or spatial relationship; perceptual or cognitive impairment; pain; neuromuscular impairment; musculoskeletal impairment; environmental barriers

Defining characteristics: inability to get bath supplies; inability to wash body or body parts; inability to obtain or get to water source; inability to regulate temperature or flow of bath water; inability to get in and out of bathroom; inability to dry body

Self-care deficit, dressing/grooming

Definition: an impaired ability to perform or complete dressing and grooming activities for oneself (see suggested functional level classification under diagnosis *Impaired Physical Mobility*)

Related factors: decreased or lack of motivation; pain; severe anxiety; perceptual or cognitive impairment; neuromuscular impairment; musculoskeletal impairment; discomfort; environmental barriers; weakness or tiredness

Defining characteristics: inability to choose clothing; inability to use assistive devices; inability to use zippers; inability to remove clothes; inability to put on socks; inability to put on clothing on upper body; impaired ability to put on or take off necessary items of clothing; impaired ability to fasten clothing; impaired ability to obtain or replace articles of clothing; inability to maintain appearance at a satisfactory level; inability to put on clothing on lower body; inability to pick up clothing; inability to put on shoes

Self-care deficit, feeding

Definition: an impaired ability to perform or complete feeding activities

Related factors: weakness or tiredness; severe anxiety; neuromuscular impairment; pain; perceptual or cognitive impairment; discomfort; environmental barriers; decreased or lack of motivation; musculoskeletal impairments

Defining characteristics: inability to swallow food; inability to prepare food for ingestion; inability to handle utensils; inability to chew food; inability to use assistive device; inability to get food onto utensil; inability to open containers; inability to manipulate food in mouth; inability to ingest food safely; inability to bring food from a receptacle to the mouth; inability to complete a meal; inability to ingest food in a socially acceptable manner; inability to pick up cup or glass; inability to ingest sufficient food

Self-care deficit, toileting

Definition: an impaired ability to perform or complete own toileting activities

Related factors: environmental barriers; weakness or tiredness; decreased or lack of motivation; severe anxiety; impaired mobility status; impaired transfer ability; musculoskeletal impairment; neuromuscular impairment; pain; perceptual or cognitive impairment

Defining characteristics: inability to manipulate clothing, unable to carry out proper toilet hygiene; unable to sit on or rise from toilet or commode; unable to get to toilet or commode; unable to flush toilet or commode

Self-esteem, chronic low

Definition: long standing negative self-evaluation/feelings about self or self-capabilities

Related factors: to be developed

Defining characteristics: rationalizes away/rejects positive feedback and exaggerates negative feedback about self (long standing or chronic); self-negating verbalization (long standing or chronic); hesitant to try new things/situations (long standing or chronic); expressions of shame/guilt (long standing or chronic); evaluates self as unable to deal with events (long standing or chronic); lack of eye contact; nonassertive/passive; frequent lack of success in work or other life events; excessively seeks reassurance; overly conforming; dependent on others' opinions; indecisive

Self-esteem, disturbance

Definition: negative self-evaluation/feelings about self or self-capabilities, which may be directly or indirectly expressed

Related factors: to be developed

Defining characteristics: grandiosity; rationalizes away/rejects positive feedback and exaggerates negative feedback about self; rationalization of personal failures; projection of blame/responsibility for problems; self-negating verbalization; expressions of shame/guilt; evaluates self as unable to deal with events; denial of problems obvious to others; hypersensitivity to slight or criticism; hesitant to try new things/situations

Self-esteem, situational low

Definition: negative self-evaluation/feelings about self that develop in response to a loss or change in an individual who previously had a positive self-evaluation

Related factors: to be developed

Defining characteristics: verbalization of negative feelings about self (e.g., helplessness, uselessness); episodic occurrence of negative self-appraisal in response to life events in a person with a previous positive self-evaluation; difficulty making decisions; evaluates self as unable to handle situations/events; expressions of shame/guilt; self-negating verbalizations

Self-mutilation, risk for
Definition: a state in which an individual is at high risk to perform an act upon the self to injure, not kill, which produces tissue damage and tension relief
Risk factors: command hallucinations; need for sensory stimuli; mentally retarded and autistic children; inability to cope with increased psychological/physiological tension in a healthy manner; history of physical, emotional, or sexual abuse; fluctuating emotions; feelings of depression, rejection, self-hatred, separation anxiety, guilt and depersonalization; dysfunctional family; clients with borderline personality disorder, especially females 16–25 years of age; clients with a history of self-injury; clients in psychotic state—frequently males in young adulthood; parental emotional deprivation; emotionally disturbed and/or battered children

Sensory/perceptual alterations (specify: auditory, gustatory, kinesthetic, olfactory, tactile, visual)
Definition: a state in which an individual experiences a change in the amount or pattering of incoming stimuli accompanied by a diminished, exaggerated, distorted or impaired response to such stimuli
Related factors: altered sensory perception; excessive environmental stimuli; psychological stress; altered sensory reception, transmission, and/or integration; insufficient environmental stimuli; biochemical imbalances for sensory distortions (e.g., illusions, hallucinations); electrolyte imbalance; biochemical imbalance
Defining characteristics: poor concentration; auditory distortions; change in usual response to stimuli; restlessness; reported or measured change in sensory acuity; irritability; disoriented in time, in place, or with people; change in problem-solving abilities; change in behavior pattern; altered communication patterns; hallucinations; visual distortions

Sexual dysfunction
Definition: a state in which an individual experiences a change in sexual function that is viewed as unsatisfying, unrewarding, inadequate
Related factors: misinformation or lack of knowledge; vulnerability; values conflict; psychosocial abuse (e.g., harmful relationships); physical abuse; lack of privacy; ineffectual or absent role models; altered body structure or function (e.g., pregnancy, recent childbirth, drugs, surgery, anomalies, disease process, trauma, radiation); lack of significant other; biopsychosocial alteration of sexuality
Defining characteristics: change of interest in self and others; conflicts involving values; inability to achieve desired satisfaction; verbalization of problem; alteration in relationship with significant other; alteration in achieving sexual satisfaction; actual or perceived limitations imposed by disease and/or therapy; seeking confirmation of desirability; alterations in achieving perceived sex role

Sexuality patterns, altered
Definition: the state in which an individual expresses concern regarding his/her sexuality
Related factors: lack of significant other; conflicts with sexual orientation or variant preferences; fear of pregnancy or of acquiring a sexually transmitted disease; impaired relationship with a significant other; ineffective or absent role models; knowledge/skill deficit about alternative responses to health-related transitions, altered body function or structure, illness or medical; lack of privacy
Defining characteristics: reported difficulties, limitations, or changes in sexual behaviors or activities

Skin integrity, impaired
Definition: a state in which an individual has altered epidermis and/or dermis.
Related factors:
External: hyperthermia or hypothermia; chemical substance; humidity; mechanical factors (e.g., shearing forces, pressure, restraint); physical immobilization; radiation; extremes in age; moisture; altered fluid status; medications
Internal: altered metabolic state; skeletal prominence; immunological deficit; developmental factors; altered sensation; altered nutritional state (e.g., obesity, emaciation); altered pigmentation; altered circulation; alterations in turgor (changes in elasticity)
Defining characteristics: invasion of body structures; destruction of skin layers (dermis); disruption of skin surface (epidermis)

Skin integrity, risk for impaired
Definition: a state in which an individual's skin is at risk of being adversely altered
Risk factors:
External: radiation; physical immobilization; mechanical factors (e.g., shearing forces, pressure, restraint); hypothermia or hyperthermia; humidity; chemical substance; excretions and/or secretions; moisture; extremes of age
Internal: medication; skeletal prominence; immunologic; developmental factors; altered sensation; altered pigmentation; altered metabolic state; altered circulation; alterations in skin turgor (changes in elasticity); alterations in nutritional state (e.g., obesity, emaciation); psychogenetic

Sleep deprivation
Definition: prolonged periods of time without sustained natural, periodic suspension of relative unconsciousness
Related factors: prolonged physical discomfort; prolonged psychological discomfort; sustained inadequate sleep hygiene; prolonged use of pharmacologic or dietary antisoporifics; aging-related sleep stage shifts; sustained circadian asynchrony; inadequate daytime activity; sustained environmental stimulation; sustained unfamiliar or uncomfortable sleep environment; nonsleep-inducing parenting practices; sleep apnea; periodic limb movement (e.g., restless leg syndrome, nocturnal myoclonus); sundowner's syndrome; narcolepsy; idiopathic central nervous system hypersomnolence; sleep walking; sleep terror; sleep-related enuresis; nightmares; familial sleep paralysis; sleep-related painful erections; dementia
Defining characteristics: daytime drowsiness; decreased ability to function; malaise; tiredness; lethargy; restlessness; irritability; heightened sensitivity to pain; listlessness; apathy; slowed reactional inability to concentrate; perceptual disorders (e.g., disturbed body sensation, delusions, feeling afloat); hallucinations; acute confusion; transient paranoia; agitated or combative; anxious; mild, fleeting nystagmus; hand tremors

Sleep pattern disturbance
Definition: time limited disruption of sleep (natural, periodic suspension of consciousness) amount and quality
Related factors:
Psychological: ruminative pre-sleep thoughts; daytime activity pattern; thinking about home; body temperature; temperament; dietary; childhood onset; inadequate sleep hygiene; sustained use of anti-sleep agents; circadian asynchrony; frequently changing sleep-wake schedule; depression; loneliness; frequent travel across time zones; daylight/darkness exposure; grief; anticipation; shift work; delayed or advanced sleep phase syndrome; loss of sleep partner, life change; preoccupation with trying to sleep; periodic gender-related hormonal shifts; biochemical agents; fear; separation from significant others; social schedule inconsistent with chronotype; aging-related sleep shifts; anxiety; medications; fear of insomnia; maladaptive conditioned wakefulness; fatigue; boredom
Environmental: noise; unfamiliar sleep furnishings; ambient temperature; humidity; lighting; other-generated awakening; excessive stimulation; physical restraint; lack of sleep privacy/control; nurse for therapeutics, monitoring, lab tests; sleep partner; noxious odors
Parental: mother's sleep-wake pattern; parent-infant interaction; mother's emotional support
Physiological: urinary urgency; wet; fever, nausea; stasis of secretions; shortness of breath; position; gastroesophageal reflux
Defining characteristics: prolonged awakenings; sleep maintenance insomnia; self-induced impairment of normal pattern; sleep onset greater than 30 minutes; early morning insomnia; awakening earlier or later than desired; verbal complaints of difficulty falling asleep; verbal complaints of not feeling well-rested; increased proportion of stage 1 sleep; dissatisfaction with sleep; less than age-normed total sleep time; three or more nighttime awakenings; decreased proportion of stages 3 and 4 sleep (e.g., hyporesponsiveness, excess sleepiness, decreased motivation); decreased proportion of REM sleep (e.g., REM rebound, hyperactivity, emotional lability, agitation and impulsivity, atypical polysomnographic features); decreased ability to function

Social interaction, impaired
Definition: the state in which an individual participates in an insufficient or excessive quantity or ineffective quality of social exchange
Related factors: knowledge/skill deficit about ways to enhance mutuality; therapeutic isolation; sociocultural dissonance; limited physical mobility; environmental barriers; communication barriers; altered thought processes; absence of available significant others or peers; self-concept disturbance

Defining characteristics: verbalized or observed inability to receive or communicate a satisfying sense of belonging, caring, interest, or shared history; verbalized or observed discomfort in social situations; observed use of unsuccessful social interaction behaviors; dysfunctional interaction with peers, family and/or others; family report of change of style or pattern of interaction

Social isolation
Definition: aloneness experienced by the individual and perceived as imposed by others and as a negative or threatened state
Related factors: alterations in mental status; inability to engage in satisfying personal relationships; unaccepted social values; unaccepted social behavior; inadequate personal resources; immature interests; factors contributing to the absence of satisfying personal relationships (e.g., delay in accomplishing developmental tasks); alterations in physical appearance; altered state of wellness
Defining characteristics:
Objective: absence of supportive significant other(s) [family, friends, group]; projects hostility in voice, behavior; withdrawn; uncommunicative; shows behavior unaccepted by dominant cultural group; seeks to be alone or exists in a subculture; repetitive, meaningless actions; preoccupation with own thoughts; no eye contact; evidence of physical/mental handicap or altered state of wellness; sad, dull affect
Subjective: expresses feeling of aloneness imposed by others; expresses feelings of rejection; inappropriate or immature interests/activities for development age/stage; inadequate or absent significant purpose in life; inability to meet expectation of others; expresses values acceptable to the subculture but unacceptable to the dominant cultural group; expresses interests inappropriate to the developmental age/stage; experiences feelings of differences from others; insecurity in public

Sorrow, chronic
Definition: a cyclical, recurring and potentially progressive pattern of pervasive sadness that is experienced [by a client (parent or caregiver, or individual with chronic illness or disability)] in response to continual loss, throughout the trajectory of an illness or disability
Related factors: death of a loved one; person experiences chronic physical or mental illness or disability such as: mental retardation, multiple sclerosis, prematurity, spina bifida or other birth defects, infertility, cancer, Parkinson's disease; person experiences one or more trigger events (e.g., crises in management of the illness, crises related to developmental stages and missed opportunities or milestones that bring comparisons with developmental, social, or personal norms); unending caregiving as a constant reminder of loss
Defining characteristics: feelings that vary in intensity, are periodic, may progress and intensify over time, and may interfere with the client's ability to reach his/her highest level of personal and social well-being; client expresses periodic, recurrent feelings of sadness; client expresses one or more of the following feelings: anger, being misunderstood, confusion, depression, disappointment, emptiness, fear, frustration, guilt/self-blame, helplessness, hopelessness, loneliness, low self-esteem, recurring loss, overwhelmed

Spiritual distress
Definition: disruption in the life principle that pervades a person's entire being and that integrates and transcends one's biological and psychosocial nature
Related factors: challenged belief and value system (e.g., due to moral/ethical implications of therapy, intense suffering); separation from religious/cultural ties
Defining characteristics: expresses concern with meaning of life/death and/or belief systems (critical); questions moral/ethical implications of therapeutic regime; description of nightmares/sleep disturbances; verbalizes inner conflict about beliefs; verbalizes concern about relationship with deity; unable to participate in usual religious practices; seeks spiritual assistance; questions meaning of suffering; questions meaning of own existence; displacement of anger toward religious representatives; anger toward God; alteration in behavior/mood evidenced by anger, crying, withdrawal, preoccupation, anxiety, hostility, apathy, etc.; gallows humor

Spiritual distress, risk for
Definition: at risk for an altered sense of harmonious connectedness with all of life and the universe in which dimensions that transcend and empower the self may be disrupted

Risk factors: energy-consuming anxiety; low self-esteem; mental illness; physical illness; blocks to self-love; poor relationships; physical or psychological stress; substance abuse; loss of loved one; natural disasters; situation losses; maturational losses; inability to forgive

Spiritual well-being, potential for enhanced

Definition: spiritual well-being is the process of an individual's developing/unfolding of mystery through harmonious interconnectedness that springs from inner strengths

Defining characteristics:

Inner strength: inner core; transcended; self-consciousness; unifying force; a sense of awareness; sacred source

Unfolding mystery: one's experience about life's purpose and meaning, mystery, uncertainty, and struggles

Harmonious interconnectedness: harmony with self, others, higher power/God, and the environment; relatedness with self, others, higher power/God, and the environment; connectedness with self, others, higher power/God, and the environment

Suffocation, risk for

Definition: accentuated risk of accidental suffocation (i.e., inadequate air available for inhalation)

Risk factors:

External: vehicle warming in closed garage; use of fuel-burning heaters not vented to outside; smoking in bed; children playing with plastic bags or inserting small objects into their mouths or noses; propped bottle placed in an infant's crib; pillow placed in an infant's crib; person who eats large mouthfuls of food; discarded or unused refrigerators or freezers without removed doors; children left unattended in bathtubs or pools; household gas leaks; low strung clothesline; pacifier hung around infant's head

Internal: reduced olfactory sensation; reduced motor abilities; cognitive or emotional difficulties; disease or injury process; lack of safety education; lack of safety precautions

Surgical recovery, delayed

Definition: an extension of the number of postoperative days required for individuals to initiate and perform on their own behalf activities that maintain life, health, and well-being

Related factors: to be developed

Defining characteristics: evidence of interrupted healing of surgical area (e.g., red, indurated, draining, immobile); loss of appetite with or without nausea; difficulty in moving about; requires help to complete self-care; fatigue; report of pain/discomfort; postpones resumption of work/employment activities; perception more time is needed to recover

Swallowing, impaired

Definition: abnormal functioning of the swallowing mechanism associated with deficits in oral, pharyngeal, or esophageal structure or function

Related factors:

Congenital deficits: upper airway anomalies; failure to thrive or protein energy malnutrition; conditions with significant hypotonia; respiratory disorders; history of tube feeding; behavioral feeding problems; self injurious behavior; neuromuscular impairment (e.g., decreased or absent gag reflex, decreased strength or excursion of muscles involved in mastication, perceptual impairment, facial paralysis); mechanical obstruction (e.g., edema, tracheostomy tube, tumor); congenital heart disease; cranial nerve involvement

Neurological problems: upper airway anomalies; laryngeal abnormalities; achalasia; gastroesophageal reflux disease; acquired anatomic defects; cerebral palsy; internal traumas; tracheal, laryngeal, esophageal defects; traumatic head injury; developmental delay; external traumas; nasal or nasopharyngeal cavity defects; oral cavity or oropharynx abnormalities; premature infants

Defining characteristics:

Pharyngeal phase impairment: altered head positions; inadequate laryngeal elevation; food refusal; unexplained fevers; delayed swallow; recurrent pulmonary infections; gurgly voice quality; nasal reflux; choking, coughing, or gagging; multiple swallows; abnormality in pharyngeal phase by swallow study

Esophageal phase impairment: heartburn or epigastric pain; acidic smelling breath; unexplained irritability surrounding mealtime; vomitus on pillow; repetitive swallowing or ruminating; regurgitation of gastric contents or wet burps; bruxism; nighttime coughing or awakening; observed evidence of difficulty in swallowing (e.g., stasis of food in oral cavity,

coughing/choking); hyperextension of head, arching during or after meals; abnormality in esophageal phase by swallow study; odynophagia; food refusal or volume limiting; complaints of "something stuck"; hematemesis; vomiting
Oral phase impairment: lack of tongue action to form bolus; weak suck resulting in inefficient nippling; incomplete lip closure; food pushed out of mouth; slow bolus formation; food falls from mouth; premature entry of bolus; nasal reflux; inability to clear oral cavity; long meals with little consumption; coughing, choking, gagging before a swallow; abnormality in oral phase of swallow study; piecemeal deglutition; lack of chewing; pooling lateral sulci; sialorrhea or drooling

Thermoregulation, ineffective
Definition: the state in which an individual's temperature fluctuates between hypothermia and hyperthermia
Related factors: aging; fluctuating environmental temperature; immaturity; trauma or illness
Defining characteristics: fluctuations in body temperature above or below the normal range; cool skin; cyanotic nail beds; flushed skin; hypertension; increased respiratory rate; pallor (moderate); piloerection; reduction in body temperature below normal range; seizures/convulsions; shivering (mild); slow capillary refill; tachycardia; warm to touch

Thought processes, altered
Definition: a state in which an individual experiences a disruption in cognitive operations and activities
Related factors: to be developed
Defining characteristics: cognitive dissonance; memory deficit/problems; inaccurate interpretation of environment; hypovigilance; hypervigilance; distractibility; egocentricity; inappropriate nonreality-based thinking

Tissue integrity, impaired
Definition: a state in which an individual experiences damage to mucous membrane, corneal, integumentary, or subcutaneous tissues. It is a state in which an individual has altered body tissue
Related factors: mechanical (e.g., pressure, shear, friction); radiation (including therapeutic radiation); nutritional deficit or excess; thermal (temperature extremes); knowledge deficit; irritants, chemical (including body excretions, secretions, medications); impaired physical mobility; altered circulation; fluid deficit or excess.
Defining characteristics: damaged or destroyed tissue (e.g., cornea, mucous membrane, integumentary, or subcutaneous)

Tissue perfusion, altered (specify type: renal, cerebral, cardiopulmonary, gastrointestinal, peripheral)
Definition: A decrease in oxygen resulting in the failure to nourish the tissues at the capillary level
Related factors: hypovolemia; interruption of flow, arterial; hypervolemia; exchange problems; interruption of flow, venous; mechanical reduction of venous and/or arterial blood flow; hypoventilation; impaired transport of the oxygen across alveolar and/or capillary membrane; mismatch of ventilation with blood flow; decreased hemoglobin concentration in blood; enzyme poisoning; altered affinity of hemoglobin for oxygen
Defining characteristics:
Renal: altered blood pressure outside of acceptable parameters; hematuria; oliguria or anuria; elevation in BUN/Creatinine ratio; skin color diminished arterial pulsations; skin color pale on elevation, color does not return on lowering of leg; slow healing of lesions; claudication; blood pressure changes in extremities; bruits
Gastrointestinal: hypoactive or absent bowel sounds; nausea; abdominal distention; abdominal pain or tenderness
Peripheral: edema; positive Homan's sign; altered skin characteristics (hair, nails, moisture); weak or absent pulses; skin discolorations; skin temperature changes; *altered sensations*
Cerebral: speech abnormalities; changes in pupillary reactions; extremity weakness or paralysis; altered mental status; difficulty in swallowing; changes in motor response; behavioral changes
Cardiopulmonary: altered respiratory rate outside of acceptable parameters; use of accessory muscles; capillary refill greater than 3 seconds; abnormal arterial blood gases; chest pain; sense of "impending doom"; bronchospasms; dyspnea; arrhythmias; nasal flaring; chest retraction

Transfer ability, impaired
Definition: limitation of independent movement between two nearby surfaces [specify level]
Suggested Functional Level Classification:
0 = is completely independent
1 = requires use of equipment or device
2 = requires help from another person for assistance, supervision, or teaching

3 = requires help from another person and equipment/device
4 = is dependent; does not participate in activity
Related factors: to be developed
Defining characteristics: impaired ability to transfer from bed to chair and chair to bed; impaired ability to transfer on or off a toilet or commode; impaired ability to transfer in and out of tub or shower; impaired ability to transfer from chair to car or car to chair; impaired ability to transfer from chair to floor or floor to chair; impaired ability to transfer from standing to floor or floor to standing

Trauma, risk for
Definition: accentuated risk of accidental tissue injury (e.g., wound, burn, fracture)
Risk factors:
External: high crime neighborhood and vulnerable clients; pot handles facing toward front of stove; knives stored uncovered; inappropriate call-for-aid mechanisms for bed-resting client; inadequately stored combustible or corrosives (e.g., matches, oily rags, lye); highly flammable children's toys or clothing; obstructed passageways; high beds; large icicles hanging from roof; nonuse or misuse of seat restraints; overexposure to sun, sun lamps, radiotherapy; overloaded electrical outlets; overloaded fuse boxes; play or work near vehicle pathways (e.g., driveways, laneways, railroad tracks); playing with fireworks or gunpowder; guns or ammunition stored unlocked; contact with rapidly moving machinery, industrial belts, or pulleys; litter or liquid spills on floors or stairways; defective appliances; bathing in very hot water (e.g., unsupervised bathing of young children); bathtub without hand grip or antislip equipment; children playing with matches, candles, cigarettes, sharp-edged toys; children riding in the front seat in car; delayed lighting of gas burner or oven; contact with intense cold; grease waste collected on stoves; driving a mechanically unsafe vehicle; driving after partaking of alcoholic beverages or drugs; driving at excessive speeds; entering unlighted rooms; experimenting with chemical or gasoline; exposure to dangerous machinery; faulty electrical plugs; frayed wires; contact with acids or alkalis; unsturdy or absent stair rails; use of unsteady ladders or chairs; use of cracked dishware or glasses; wearing plastic apron or flowing clothes around open flame; unscreened fires or heaters; unsafe window protection in homes with young children; sliding on coarse bed linen or struggling within bed restraints; use of thin or worn potholders; misuse of necessary headgear for motorized cyclists or young children carried on adult bicycles; potential igniting gas leaks; unsafe road or road-crossing conditions; slippery floors (e.g., wet or highly waxed); smoking in bed or near oxygen; snow or ice collected on stairs, walkways; unanchored electric wires; unanchored rugs, driving without necessary visual aids
Internal: lack of safety education; insufficient finances to purchase safety equipment or effect repairs; history of previous trauma; lack of safety precautions; poor vision; reduced temperature and/or tactile sensation; balancing difficulties; cognitive or emotional difficulties; reduced large or small muscle coordination; weakness; reduced hand-eye coordination.

Unilateral neglect
Definition: the state in which an individual is perceptually unaware of and inattentive to one side of the body
Related factors: effects of disturbed perceptual abilities (e.g., hemianopsia); neurologic illness or trauma; one-sided blindness
Defining characteristics: consistent inattention to stimuli on an affected side; does not look toward affected side; positioning and/or safety precautions in regard to the affected side; inadequate self-care; leaves food on plate on the affected side

Urinary elimination, altered
Definition: the state in which an individual experiences a disturbance in urine-elimination.
Related factors: urinary tract infection; anatomical obstruction; multiple causality; sensory motor impairment
Defining characteristics: incontinence; urgency; nocturia; hesitancy; frequency; dysuria; retention

Urinary retention
Definition: the state in which the individual experiences incomplete emptying of bladder
Related factors: blockage; high urethral pressure caused by weak detrusor; inhibition of reflex arc; strong sphincter
Defining characteristics: bladder distention; small, frequent voiding or absence of urine output; dribbling; dysuria; overflow incontinence; residual urine; sensation of bladder fullness

Ventilation, inability to sustain spontaneous

Definition: a state in which the response pattern of decreased energy reserves results in an individual's inability to maintain breathing adequate to support life

Related factors: respiratory muscle fatigue; metabolic factors

Defining characteristics: dyspnea; increased metabolic rate; increased pCO_2; increased restlessness; increased hear rate; decreased tidal volume; decreased pO_2; decreased cooperation; apprehension; decreased SaO_2; increased use of accessory muscles

Ventilatory weaning response, dysfunctional

Definition: a state in which an individual cannot adjust to lowered levels of mechanical ventilator support, which interrupts and prolongs the weaning process

Related factors:

Psychological: patient perceived inefficacy about the ability to wean; powerlessness; anxiety: moderate to severe; knowledge deficit of the weaning process; patient role; hopelessness; fear; decreased motivation; decreased self-esteem; insufficient trust in the nurse

Situational: uncontrolled episodic energy demands or problems; adverse environment (e.g., noisy, active environment, negative events in the room, low nurse-patient ratio, extended nurse absence from bedside, unfamiliar nursing staff); history of multiple unsuccessful weaning attempts; history of ventilator dependence greater than 1 week; inappropriate pacing of diminished ventilator support; inadequate social support.

Defining characteristics:

Severe: deterioration in arterial blood gases from current baseline; respiratory rate increases significantly from baseline; increase from baseline blood pressure (>20 mm Hg); agitation; increase from baseline heart rate (>20 beats/min); paradoxical abdominal breathing; adventitious breath sounds, audible airway secretions; cyanosis; decreased level of consciousness; full respiratory accessory muscle use; shallow, gasping breaths; profuse diaphoresis; discoordinated breathing with the ventilator

Moderate: slight increase from baseline blood pressure (<20 mm Hg); baseline increase in respiratory rate (<5 breaths/min); slight increase from baseline heart rate (<20 beats/min); pale, slight cyanosis; slight respiratory accessory muscle use; inability to respond to coaching; inability to cooperate; apprehension; color changes; decreased air entry on auscultation; diaphoresis; eye widening (wide-eyed look); hypervigilance to activities

Mild: warmth; restlessness; slight increase of respiratory rate from baseline; queries about possible machine malfunction; expressed feelings of increased need for oxygen; fatigue; increased concentration on breathing; breathing discomfort

Violence: directed at others, risk for

Definition: behaviors in which an individual demonstrates that he/she can be physically, emotionally, and/or sexually harmful to others

Risk factors: history of violence against others (e.g., hitting someone, kicking someone, spitting at someone, biting someone, attempted rape, rape, sexual molestation, urinating/defecating on a person); history of violence of threats (e.g., verbal threats against property, verbal threats against person, social threats, cursing, threatening notes/letters, threatening gestures, sexual threats); history of violent antisocial behavior (e.g., stealing, insistent borrowing, insistent demands for privileges, insistent interruption of meetings, refusal to eat, refusal to take medication, ignoring instructions); history of violence, indirect (e.g., tearing off clothes, ripping objects off walls, writing on walls, urinating on floor, defecating on floor, stamping feet, temper tantrum, running in corridors, yelling, throwing objects, breaking a window, slamming doors, sexual advances); other factors: neurological impairment (e.g., positive EEG, CAT, or MRI, head trauma, positive neurological findings, seizure disorders); cognitive impairment (e.g., learning disabilities, attention deficit disorder, decreased intellectual functioning); history of childhood abuse; history of witnessing family violence; cruelty to animals; firesetting; prenatal and perinatal complications/abnormalities; history of drug/alcohol abuse; pathological intoxication; psychotic symptomatology (e.g., auditory, visual, command hallucinations; paranoid delusions; loose, rambling of illogical thought processes); motor vehicle offenses (e.g., frequent traffic violations, use of a motor vehicle to release anger); suicidal behavior, impulsivity; availability and/or possession of weapon(s); body language; rigid posture, clenching of fists and jaw, hyperactivity, pacing, breathlessness, threatening stances.

Violence: self-directed, risk for

Definition: behaviors in which an individual demonstrates that he/she can be physically, emotionally and/or sexually harmful to self

Risk factors: age 15–19; age over 45; marital status (single, widowed, divorced); employment (unemployed, recent job loss/failure); occupation (executive, administrator/owner of business, professional, semi-skilled worker); conflictual interpersonal relationships; family background (chaotic or conflictual, history of suicide); sexual orientation (bisexual [active], homosexual [inactive]); physical health (hypochondriac, chronic or terminal illness); mental health (severe depression, psychosis, severe personality disorder, alcoholism or drug abuse); emotional status (hopelessness, despair, increased anxiety, panic, anger, hostility); history of multiple suicide attempts; suicidal ideation (frequent, intense, prolonged); suicidal plan (clear and specific; lethality: method and availability of destructive means); personal resources (poor achievement, poor insight, affect unavailable and poorly controlled); social resources (poor rapport, socially isolated, unresponsive family); verbal clues (e.g., talking about death, better off without me, asking questions about lethal dosages of drugs); behavioral clues (e.g., writing forlorn love notes, directing angry messages at a significant other who has rejected the person, giving away personal items, taking out a large life insurance policy); people who engage in autoerotic sexual acts

Walking, impaired

Definition: limitation of independent movement within the environment on foot [specify level]

Suggested Functional Level Classification:

0 = is completely independent

1 = requires use of equipment or device

2 = requires help from another person for assistance, supervision, or teaching

3 = requires help from another person and equipment/device

4 = is dependent; does not participate in activity

Related factors: to be developed

Defining characteristics: impaired ability to climb stairs; impaired ability to walk required distances; impaired ability to walk on an incline or decline; impaired ability to walk on uneven surfaces; impaired ability to navigate curbs

Appendix B

INVASIVE PROCEDURES	DATE	SITE	DATE	RESPIRATORY THERAPY	START DATE	MEDICATIONS	DOSAGE	METHOD	INTERVAL	HOURS
A LINE				TYPE						
SWAN-GANZ				O₂						
CVP LINE										
TRIPLE LUMEN										
®ATRIAL CATHETER										
PORTACATH										
NG TUBE										
SHUNT / ACCESS				DATE	DIAGNOSTICS					
WOUND DRAIN #1					I & Oq					
WOUND DRAIN #2					C & Aq					
URINARY CATHETER					FUNDAL √q					
CHEST TUBE #1					DTR'Sq					
CHEST TUBE #2					LOCHIA √q					
PACEMAKER P/T										
FIXED / DEMAND										
V / A-V SEQ.				DATE	ACTIVITIES					
OUTPUT					CBR					
PACING THRESHOLD					BRP					
SENS. RATE					AMB					
A / V INT.					W/C					
TRACHEOSTOMY / SIZE					TCDBq					
DIALYSIS H/P					POSITIONING					
COLOSTOMY					ROMq					

IV THERAPY

FLUID / TYPE	RATE / HR.	SITE	DATE INS.	DRESSING CHANGE	TUBING CHANGE	INSERTION SITE CHANGE

DATE	VITAL SIGNS	START DATE	PRN MEDICATION
	TPRq		
	BPq		
	NEURO √q		

DATE	SPECIAL NEEDS	DATE	TREATMENTS
	ORIENTED		SITZ BATH
	DISORIENTED/HIGH RISK		TED HOSE
	R/O PPD		
	SUICIDE PRECAUTIONS		
	SEIZURE PRECAUTIONS		

DATE	NURSING TREATMENTS AND SPECIAL PROCEDURES

KARDEX REVIEWED PRIOR TO TRANSFER

BY DR.	DATE
SIGNATURE	
BY DR.	DATE
SIGNATURE	
BY DR.	DATE
SIGNATURE	

APPENDIX B–1 The Kardex is a quick reference tool, sometimes used during report. Reprinted with permission from Conroe Regional Medical Center Hospital, Conroe, Texas.

(continues)

SUNDAY	MONDAY	TUESDAY	WEDNESDAY
DATE	DATE	DATE	DATE

THURSDAY	FRIDAY	SATURDAY	DAILY & TIMED
DATE	DATE	DATE	

COMMUNICATIONS

ISOLATION: TYPE _____

HIGH RISK PATIENT   YES ☐   NO ☐

NOTIFY IN EMERGENCY

NAME _____   RELATIONSHIP _____   ADDRESS _____   PHONE NO. _____

MONITOR	CODE BLUE	DATE	D.N.R.	DATE	PER:	PHYSICIAN

ALLERGIES

	DIET		HEIGHT	WEIGHT

	SURGERY		DATE

DATE OF ADMIT	DIAGNOSIS		SEX	AGE	PRIMARY PHYSICIAN
ROOM NO.	PATIENTS NAME				

CONSULTS

GEST _____ GR _____ PARA _____ AB _____ ANESTH _____

EPIS _____ LAC _____ RUBELLA IMMUNE/NON-IMMUNE

MOTHERS BLOOD TYPE _____ RH _____ BOTTLE/BREAST _____

BABYS BLOOD TYPE _____ WT _____ SEX _____ APGAR _____

DELIVERY DATE _____ TIME _____

NS-34 (REV. 9/86)

Patient History and General Information ☐ ID bracelet placed

Nursing Unit: _____ Date: _____ Time: _____ Mode: ☐ Ambulatory ☐ Wheelchair ☐ Stretcher ☐ Ambulance

Origin: ☐ Home ☐ Dr's Office ☐ ER ☐ Nursing Home ☐ Other_____ Marital Status: ☐ Single ☐ Married ☐ Divorced ☐ Widowed

Information Provided by ☐ Patient ☐ Family/SO_____ ☐ No Available Informant at Time of Admission ☐ Transfer Form

GENERAL

Chief complaint / Reason for hospitalization: (State in patient's own words) _____

Summarize current illness episode _____

_____

Initial vital signs   T_____ P_____ R_____   BP: RA _____ LA _____   Height: _____

☐ TYMPANIC ☐ ORAL ☐ RECTAL ☐ AXILLARY   ☐ LYING ☐ STANDING ☐ SITTING   Weight: stated_____ actual_____

MEDICAL HISTORY

Family History

☐ Diabetes ☐ Asthma ☐ COPD ☐ Heart Disease ☐ High BP ☐ Cancer ☐ Kidney Disease ☐ Seizures

Patient History

☐ Diabetes ☐ Asthma ☐ COPD ☐ Heart Disease ☐ High BP ☐ Cancer ☐ Kidney Disease ☐ Seizures ☐ Hepatitis ☐ Glaucoma

Other medical and surgical history _____

_____

Patient Allergy History   ☐ No Known Allergies   ☐ If Allergy bracelet placed   ☐ Potential for Injury, Allergy

☐ Food _____

☐ Medications _____   ☐ Activate Latex Avoidance Practices

☐ Latex (Rubber) _____

☐ Dyes/Contrast Media _____

☐ Other _____

☐ Anesthesia Reaction _____ ☐ Transfusion Reaction _____

CURRENT MEDICATIONS

Name / Dose / Time *Include Herbs and Botanicals*	Last Dose	Code	Name / Dose / Time *Include Herbs and Botanicals*	Last Dose	Code	CODES
						A - Sent home with family
						B - At Bedside
						C - Not Brought with Patient
						D - In Pharmacy
						☐ Pt. instructed not to take own meds

Tobacco / Drug Usage	Alcohol Consumption

VALUABLES

	Home	Safe	Pt	N/A		Home	Safe	Pt	N/A
Wallet	☐	☐	☐	☐	Prosthesis	☐	☐	☐	☐
$_____	☐	☐	☐	☐	Jewelry	☐	☐	☐	☐
Artificial Eye	☐	☐	☐	☐	Clothing	☐	☐	☐	☐
Hearing Aid	☐	☐	☐	☐	Wheelchair	☐	☐	☐	☐
Glasses	☐	☐	☐	☐	Cane/Walker	☐	☐	☐	☐
Contacts	☐	☐	☐	☐	Brace	☐	☐	☐	☐
Upper Dent.	☐	☐	☐	☐	Crutches	☐	☐	☐	☐
Lower Dent.	☐	☐	☐	☐	Other	☐	☐	☐	☐

Patient / SO acknowledges that Conroe Regional Medical Center shall not be liable for loss or damage of any money, jewelry, documents, clothing or other personal property of patients or visitors unless deposited for safekeeping in the hospital safe.

Patient Signature _____

Staff Signature _____

Date	Time

Data Collector's Signature _____ RN/LVN

PATIENT ORIENTATION TO ENVIRONMENT

Equipment Instructions:

☐ Bed   ☐ Call Light   ☐ Phone   ☐ Temp Control   ☐ Siderails

☐ TV   ☐ Monitors   ☐ IV Pump   ☐ O2 Safety   ☐ Admit Kit

☐ Bathroom Call Light   ☐ Mealtimes   ☐ Isolation Procedures (if applicable)

Rights and Responsibilities Instructions:

☐ Smoking Policy & Areas   ☐ Visiting Hours   ☐ Patient Handbook

RIGHTS AND RESPONSIBILITIES

☐ Patient has a Directive to Physician / Medical Power of Attorney

___ Copy is on front of chart

___ Requested to provide the hospital with a copy   ☐ Advance Directive Follow up Copy

Medical Power of Attorney Name   Tele #

☐ Patient has not executed an Advance Directive

___ Patient handbook info provided / discussed in registration

___ Patient handbook info provided / discussed on the unit   ☐ Advance Directive Follow up Execute

___ Patient wants assistance to execute one

☐ Patient unable / unwilling to discuss at time of admission to the unit   ☐ Advance Directive Follow up Info

☐ Family unavailable at time of admission to the unit

Conroe Regional Medical Center

| ADMISSION ASSESSMENT |

PATIENT IDENTIFICATION

NS-102 (REV. 02/00)

(continues)

APPENDIX B-2 Admission Assessment Form.

Reprinted with permission from Conroe Regional Medical Center Hospital, Conroe, Texas.

(continued)

Biophysical Psychosocial Assessment (completed by RN)

NORM	VARIANCE	PATIENT PROBLEM / NSG DIAGNOSIS
Neurological Assessment Alert and oriented to person, place and time. Behavior appropriate to situation. Pupils equal and reactive to light. Active ROM of all extremities and symmetry of strength. No Parasthesia. ☐ ALL PARAMETERS WNL	DISORIENTED ☐ Time ☐ Person ☐ Place PUPILS ☐ Non Reactive R__ L __ ☐ Sluggish R__ L __ ☐ Unequal ☐ Pinpoint R__ L __ ☐ Dilated R__ L __ SENSORY MOTOR IMPAIRMENT ☐ Speech ☐ Swallowing ☐ Visual ☐ Headaches ☐ Seizures ☐ Gait disturbance ☐ Unequal hand grasp ☐ Numbness ☐ Tingling	☐ Confusion ☐ Acute ☐ Chronic ☐ Thought Processes, alteration ☐ Communication, impaired, verbal ☐ Swallowing, impaired ☐ Peripheral Neurovascular, alteration ☐ Tissue Perfusion, alteration ☐ Sensory Perception, alteration
Cardiovascular Assessment Regular Radial pulse. Capillary Refill Time < 3 sec. Peripheral pulses palpable. No edema. No calf tenderness. ☐ ALL PARAMETERS WNL	☐ Rhythm irregular ☐ Tachycardia > 100 ☐ Bradycardia < 60 ☐Telemetry Number _____Rhythm _____ BP_____ ☐ Hypertension ☐ Hypotension ☐ Chest Pain EDEMA ☐ Feet/Ankles R__ L __ ☐ Pitting + _____ PULSES ☐ Abnormal Location _____	☐ Activity, intolerance ☐ Fluid Volume, deficit ☐ Fluid Volume, excess ☐ Tissue Perfusion, alteration ☐
Respiratory Assessment Regular, non labored. Breath sounds clear and equal all lobes. Respirations 12 - 20 per minute. Sputum clear, nailbeds and mucus membranes pink. ☐ ALL PARAMETERS WNL	COUGH ☐ Non Productive ☐ Sputum _____ BREATH SOUNDS ☐ Diminished R__ L __ ☐ Rhonchi R__L __ ☐ Wheezes R__ L__ ☐ Crackles R__ L __ ☐ Dyspnea ☐ Apnea ☐ Tachypnea ___ ☐ Uneven Chest Movement ☐ ET Tube ☐ Trach ☐ Vent ☐ O2 Mask ☐ O2L ___ O2 Sat ___	☐ Airway Clearance, ineffective ☐ Breathing Pattern, ineffective ☐ Tissue Perfusion, alteration ☐

Gastrointestinal Assessment
Abdomen soft, non distended, non tender. Bowel sounds present in 4 quadrants. Bowel movements within own normal patterns and consistency.
☐ ALL PARAMETERS WNL
	BOWEL SOUNDS ☐ Absent ☐ Hypoactive ☐ Hyperactive
	COMPLAINTS ☐ Constipation ☐ Flatus ☐ Nausea ☐ Vomiting
	    ☐ Increased Thirst ☐ Laxative Dependence
	ABDOMEN ☐ Distended ☐ Tender ☐ Rebound ☐ Hard
	TUBES ☐ NGT ☐ Feeding Tube ☐JP Drain ☐ Hernovac
	    ☐ Tube ☐ Gastrojejunostomy ☐ Colostomy
	    ☐ Ileostomy ☐ Other_____
		☐ Bowel Elimination, alteration
		☐ Diarrhea ☐ Constipation
		☐ Incontinence
		☐ Nutrition, alteration
		☐ Tissue Perfusion, alteration
		☐

Integumentary Assessment Skin color uniform within patient's norm. Smooth, soft, warm, dry, intact. Turgor skin lifts easily and snaps back immediately on release. Mucus membranes moist, intact, pink. Hygiene good. ☐ ALL PARAMETERS WNL	SKIN APPEARANCE ☐ Pale ☐ Cyanotic ☐ Dusky ☐ Mottled ☐ Flushed ☐ Jaundiced ☐ Other ☐ Hygiene Inadequate SKIN TEMP / CHARACTER ☐ Hot ☐ Cold ☐ Clammy ☐ Moist ☐ Turgor Sluggish / Poor ☐ Very Dry MUCUS MEMBRANES ☐ Dry ☐ Blistered ☐ Cracking CONDITION ☐ Impairment (see Dermal Injury Section)	☐ Skin Integrity, Impaired ☐ Tissue Integrity, impaired ☐ Oral Mucus Membrane, alteration ☐ Body Temperature, alteration ☐ Tissue Perfusion, alteration ☐
Musculoskeletal Assessment Absence of joint swelling and tenderness. Normal ROM of all joints. No muscle weakness. Surrounding tissues show no evidence of inflammation, nodules, nail changes, ulcerations or rashes. No deformity. ☐ ALL PARAMETERS WNL	☐ Joint Swelling / Tenderness ☐ Immobile ☐Paralysis ☐ Deformity ☐ Atrophy ☐ Contracture HOMANS POSITIVE Right ☐ Absent Left ☐ Absent ☐ Present ☐ Present	☐ Physical Mobility, impaired ☐ Peripheral Neurovascular, alteration ☐ Tissue Perfusion, alteration ☐
Genitourinary Assessment Able to empty bladder without dysuria. Bladder not distended after voiding. Urine clear and yellow to amber. Continent of Urine. No appliances used. ☐ ALL PARAMETERS WNL	☐ Hemodialysis ☐ Peritoneal Dialysis ☐ Urostomy ☐ Foley # URINE Color_____ ☐ Cloudy ☐ Sediment ☐ Frequency ☐ Burning ☐ Incontinent ☐ Bladder Distention / Retention ☐ Hematuria ☐ Nocturia ☐ Anuria ☐ In and Out Cath Pt ___ Family ___ _____	☐ Urinary Elimination, alteration ☐ Retention ☐ Incontinence ☐ Tissue Perfusion, alteration ☐
Reproductive / Sexuality If female, no vaginal bleeding, discharge or lesions. Normal menstrual periods. If male, no prostrate problems, penile bleeding, lesions or discharge. No complaints of sexual dysfunction. ☐ ALL PARAMETERS WNL	☐ Discharge color _____ amount _____ ☐ Unusual Bleeding ☐ Pain ☐ Diagnosis may affect sexuality ☐ Pregnant ☐ Post partum ☐ Breastfeeding _____	☐ Sexual dysfunction ☐ Sexual Pattern, impaired ☐ Body Image, disturbance ☐
Psycho / Social Assessment Behavior apropriate to situation. Cooperative congruent affect. Responds appropriately to all questions. ☐ ALL PARAMETERS WNL	☐ Flat Affect ☐ Lack of eye contact ☐ Withdrawn ☐Agitated ☐ Crying ☐ Uncooperative ☐ Anxious ☐ Irritable ☐ Nervous ☐ Combative ☐ Threatening ☐ Ineffective Grieving o Unable to Cope ☐ Family Issues / Dysfunction	☐ Anxiety, fear ☐ Coping, ineffective ☐ Grieving, anticipatory ☐ Powerlessness ☐

RN INITIALS _____

Conroe
Regional Medical Center

PATIENT IDENTIFICATION

ADMISSION ASSESSMENT

NS-102 p.2 (REV. 02/00)

(continues)

(continued)

Biophysical Psychosocial Assessment

	PATIENT PROBLEM/NSG DIAGNOSIS

Pain Assessment
Do you have pain now? ☐ Yes ☐ No
Have you had pain in the last several weeks or months? ☐ Yes ☐ No
If Yes, to any of the above questions fill in information below.
  1. Pain Location _____
    _____
  2. Pain Description ☐ Dull ☐ Sharp ☐ Cramping ☐ Other _____
  3. Pain Intensity Adult Pain Scale   No Pain 0 1 2 3 4 5 6 7 8 9 10 Worst Pain
  4. Duration ☐ Constant ☐ Intermittent ☐ Other _____
  5. What helps the pain _____
    _____
  6. What aggravates the pain _____

☐ Pain
☐ Pain, chronic
☐

Activities of Daily Living Assessment
ADL Needs
Hygiene ☐ self ☐ assist ☐ dependent
Activity ☐ self ☐ assist ☐ dependent
Nutrition ☐ self ☐ assist ☐ dependent
Toileting ☐ self ☐ assist ☐ dependent
Sleep ☐ sleeps well at night
    ☐ does not sleep well   What helps sleep?_____

Sensory Deficits
☐ Vision _____
☐ Hearing _____
☐ Speech _____
☐ Other _____

Assistive Device Use
☐ Cane ☐ Walker ☐ Wheelchair ☐ Bedside Commode ☐ Prosthesis
☐ Other_____

☐ Self Care, deficit
☐ Physical Mobility, impaired
☐ Activity, intolerance
☐ Sleep Pattern, disturbance
☐ Sensory Perception, alteration
☐ Communication, impaired verbal
☐

Cultural Spiritual Assessment
1. Are there any spiritual, traditional, ethnic, or cultural practice that you need to be part of your care
  ☐ Yes ☐ No
2. Is there any way the hospital can assist you with your religious / spiritual practices
  ☐ Yes ☐ No
3. Would you like to be visited by the hospital chaplain ☐ Yes ☐ No

☐ Spiritual, distress
☐ Cultural, distress
☐ Grieving, anticipatory
☐

Notify Chaplain
Notification Initials _____

PATIENT AND FAMILY EDUCATION NEEDS / READINESS ASSESSMENT

Information Provided by ☐ Patient ☐ Family / SO ☐ No Available Informant at Time of Admission
1. **Literacy / Level of Education**   Can Read ☐ Yes ☐ No   Can Write ☐ Yes ☐ No
  Highest Level of Education _____
2. **Language** ☐ English ☐ Spanish ☐Other_____ Proficient in English ☐ Yes ☐ No
  Translator needed ☐Yes ☐ No
3. **Learning Barriers** ☐ None Identified ☐ Language ☐ Memory ☐ Vision ☐ Hearing ☐ Emotional
  ☐ Ability to grasp concepts and respond ☐ Motor Skills Impairment ☐ Other _____
4. **Concerns / Needs** ☐ None Identified ☐ First hospital visit ☐ Access to community resources
  ☐ Financial concerns ☐ Religious considerations ☐ School age children education needs
  ☐ Other _____
5. **Motivation** ☐ Wants to learn ☐ Uninterested, distracted or uncooperative ☐ Denies need
  ☐ Other _____
6. **Methods** Patient/Family says they learn best by ☐ Reading booklets, information sheets
  ☐ One to one discussions ☐ Hands on practice
  ☐ Other/Explain _____
7. **Type of Education** Do you or your family need information about
  ☐ No information specified ☐ Disease process ☐ Activity ☐ Medical Devices / Equipment ☐ Diet
  ☐ Current Medications / Drug Food Interactions ☐ Other _____

☐ Knowledge Deficit
R/T _____

☐ Noncompliance

☐ Communication, impaired
  Language _____

RN INITIALS

Conroe
Regional Medical Center

PATIENT IDENTIFICATION

ADMISSION ASSESSMENT

(continues)

(continued)
Safety Risk Assessment

B = burn
C = contusion
D = decubitus
E = erythema
I = incision
L = laceration
P = petechiae
R = rash
S = scar

Left Foot   **Right Foot**

Risk for Dermal Injury

☐ Skin Integrity, impairment risk for score 2 or >

☐ Skin Integrity Impaired

Location _____
Description _____
_____
_____

Location _____
Description _____
_____

Location _____
Description _____
_____

	0	1	2	Score
Mobility	Independent	Required Assistance	Total Assistance	
Continence	Continent	Occasional Incontinence	Incontinent	
Nutrition	> 90% diet	50-90% diet	< 50% diet	
Skin Integrity	Intact	Stage I or II Pressure Sore	Stage III, IV or Multi-pressure Sore	
Old Pressure Sores/Scars	No old scars	Scars over 1 Bony Prominence	Scar over 2 Bony Prominence	
Contractures/ Fractures	No contractures or fractures	Contracture 1 Extremity or Fracture	Contracture >2 Extremities; Fracture Pelvis; Non-Healed Amputation	

Total _____

Age
☐ Sixty Years of Age or Older — 2
Medications
Anesthesia, Diuretics, Laxatives, Narcotics, CNS Depressants, Hypertensives, Insulin
☐ Uses one or more no adverse effects — 1
☐ Uses one or more with adverse effects — 2
Mobility
☐ Exhibits pattern of gait disturbance — 5
☐ Needs assist to toilet or transfer to chair — 5
Mentation
☐ Unable to comprehend instruction, use the call button or ask for assistance — 10
☐ Unable to make purposeful decisions — 10
Sensory Deficits
☐ Has impaired hearing, sight or speech — 3
History of falling
☐ Hx of orthostatic hypotension or seizures — 5
☐ Other reason _____ — 5

Total _____

Risk for Fall

☐ Injury, potential for fall for score 4 or >

TB RISK

☐ Hemoptysis   ☐ Productive Cough > 3 wks   ☐ Night Sweats   ☐ Weight Loss / Fever   ☐ None
*If any of these symptoms   Initiate Airborne Precautions and Alert MD for Follow-up

Risk for TB

☐ Infection, potential TB

DOMESTIC VIOLENCE

1. Do you currently feel unsafe at home? ☐ Yes ☐ No Why?_____
2. Have you been afraid, threatened or injured by anyone within the last year? o Yes o No
3. Have you been hit, slapped, kicked, forced to engage in unwanted sexual acts, or otherwise hurt by someone in the last year?
   ☐ Yes ☐ No_____

Risk for Domestic Violence
☐ Activate Hospital Protocol
☐ Injury, potential for abuse

RN INITIALS

Conroe
Regional Medical Center

PATIENT IDENTIFICATION

ADMISSION ASSESSMENT

NS- 102 p.4 (REV.02/00)

(continues)

(continued)

Multidisciplinary Screens

NUTRITION

	SCORE	
Usual Diet _____		If score = or > 2
☐ Difficulty with any of the following > 1 week		Notify Dietitian
☐ Vomiting ☐ Diarrhea ☐ Swallowing ☐ Chewing / Unable to eat	2	
☐ Unplanned weight loss > 10 lb. in past 4 months	8	Notification initials: ____
☐ Diagnosis of malnutrition / malabsorption	8	
☐ Surgery this admission or within the past 30 days if 65 years or older	2	
☐ Patient / family request diet education related to patient's modified diet of:_____	1	
TOTAL: _____		

DIABETES

	SCORE	
☐ New diagnosis IDDM	2	If score = or > 1
☐ New diagnosis NIDDM	1	Notify Diabetes Educator
☐ New insulin start	2	
☐ Gestational	2	If score = or > than 2
☐ Recurrent hypoglycemia	1	Request MD Order
☐ DKA or HHNK	2	
☐ Recurrent ER visits for DM	1	Notification initials: ____
TOTAL: _____		

SPEECH PATHOLOGY

	SCORE	
If ☐ Onset of the below criteria is a result of this illness or within 30 days of admission	1	If score = or > than 2
And any one or more of the following		Notify Speech Pathology
☐ Difficulty in making self understood or difficulty in understanding others	1	
☐ Patient/family reported or clinically observed choking or coughing while eating or drinking	1	
☐ Patient/family reported or clinically observed change in voice quality/teary eyes/nasal drainage after eating	1	Notification initials: ____
☐ Recent significant weight loss, dehydration or pneumonia	1	
☐ New laryngectomy or tracheostomy	1	
☐ Patient admitted with order for thickened liquids	1	
TOTAL: _____		

PT/OT

	SCORE	
If ☐ The onset of the below criteria is a result of this illness or within 30 days of admission	1	If score = or > than 3
☐ Patient / Family demonstrates potential ability to participate in rehab	1	Notify PT / OT
And any one or more of the following		
☐ Impaired functional mobility (gait transfer or bed mobility) and/or a potential for injury	1	
☐ Difficulty in performing ADLs (feeding, dressing, grooming)	1	
☐ Difficulty in management of pain / stress	1	Notification initials: ____
☐ Patient/family could benefit from splinting, positional or equipment management	1	
☐ Potential physical / occupational therapy related discharge needs	1	
TOTAL: _____		

DISCHARGE PLANNING

	SCORE	
Patient lives: ☐ alone ☐ with spouse ☐ with other family		If score is < than 5
☐ assisted / extended care facility_____		Notify Case Management in Meditech
Who can help after discharge: Name: _____ Relationship: _____		
Telephone #: _____		If score = or > than 5
Receiving these services ☐ Home Health - Agency:_____		Notify Case Management in Meditech and
prior to admission: ☐ Durable Medical Equipment - Provider:_____		voicemail Hotline (# on call schedule)
☐ Hospice - Provider:_____		
☐ Return to prior living situation unlikely	2	
☐ Unable to identify any assistance for after discharge at this time	2	
☐ Home Health Services and / or Durable Medical Equipment need anticipated at discharge	2	Notification initials:
☐ Skilled Nursing Facility or Inpatient Rehabilitation anticipated at discharge	2	
☐ Nursing Home Placement anticipated at discharge	2	☐ Complex Discharge
☐ Food, Clothing or Shelter needs identified	2	Needs
☐ Suspected Abuse or Neglect (follow hospital policy for reporting)	5	
☐ Positive Drug Screen with delivery	5	
☐ Desires an adoption plan	5	
☐ Discharge anticipated in less than 72 yours with any of the above items checked	3	
TOTAL: _____		

DATE ___ TIME ___ ADMISSION ___ RN SIGNATURE ___

Conroe
Regional Medical Center

PATIENT IDENTIFICATION

ADMISSION ASSESSMENT

NS-102 p. 5 (REV.02/00)

Date of Discharge	Time of Discharge	Mode of Discharge					Accom. by:			
		☐ Ambulatory ☐ Wheelchair ☐ Stretcher ☐ Ambulance					_____			

Belongings sent with patient or family ☐ Yes ☐ No	Personal medications sent with patient or family ☐ Yes ☐ No	Prescription sent with patient ☐ Yes ☐ No	Temp	P	R	BP

Discharge Destination	Transfer Information Sent
☐ Home ☐ AMA ☐ Facility_____ ☐ Other_____	☐ Yes ☐ No

Special Instructions

Patient Assessment and Health Status

	Yes No		Yes No		Yes No
Afebrile_____	☐ ☐	Hygiene:		Skin Intact_____	☐ ☐
Able to Live Independently____	☐ ☐	Self Care_____	☐ ☐	Eating Well_____	☐ ☐
Pain Controlled_____	☐ ☐	Assist_____	☐ ☐	Adequate Hydration_____	☐ ☐
Oriented_____	☐ ☐	Total Care_____	☐ ☐		
Appropriate Behavior_____	☐ ☐	Adequate Elimination_____	☐ ☐		
Functions Independently_____	☐ ☐				

Additional Comments

	Nurse Signature	Date

Instructions

Diet
☐ No Restrictions

Activity
☐ No Restrictions

Special Equipment/Treatment
☐ No Restrictions

Discharge Medications (Name, Amount, Special Instructions)
☐ No Meds ☐ Rx Given

Special Instructions/Discharge Summary

☐ Pt. or Caregiver given instructions about and counseled on potential for drug-food interactions.

Physician Follow-Up Appointment	Outpatient Visit

Referral
☐ None Required

I have received all personal belongings. I have received a copy and understand the above instructions.	PATIENT IDENTIFICATION
_____ Signature/Responsible Party	
_____ Physician/Nurse Signature Date	

Discharge Assessment/Instructions

N5411 07/98 (RC# 4602080)

APPENDIX B−3 Discharge Assessment Forms.
Reprinted with permission from Conroe Regional Medical Center Hospital, Conroe, Texas.

CONROE REGIONAL MEDICAL CENTER

PATIENT CARE RECORD - OBSERVATIONS

DATE: _____

PATIENT I.D. PLATE

VITAL SIGNS

HOURS	NEURO VITAL SIGNS				PULSES		OBSTETRICAL				IV	B P :00	H R :00	R E S P :00	T E M P :00	B P :15	H R :15	R E S P :15	T E M P :15	B P :30	H R :30	R E S P :30	T E M P :30	B P :45	H R :45	R E S P :45	T E M P :45
	GCS MOTOR	PUPILS ® Ⓛ	EXTREM. R.A. / R.L.	L.A. / L.L.	R.A. / R.L.	L.A. / L.L.	BREASTS	FUNDUS/PLACEMENT	LOCHIA	PERINEUM	SITE CHECK																
7A																											
8A																											
9A																											
10A																											
11A																											
12N																											
1P																											
2P																											
3P																											
4P																											
5P																											
6P																											
7P																											
8P																											
9P																											
10P																											
11P																											
12M																											
1A																											
2A																											
3A																											
4A																											
5A																											
6A																											

GLASGOW COMA SCALE

Eyes	Open	Spontaneously	4
		To verbal command	3
		To pain	2
		No response	1

	To verbal command	Obeys	6
Best motor response	To painful stimulus	Localizes Pain	5
		Flexion–Withdrawal	4
		Flexion–abnormal (decorticate rigidity)	3
		Extension (decerebrate rigidity)	2
		No response	1

Best verbal response	Oriented and converses	5
	Disoriented and converses	4
	Inappropriate words	3
	Incomprehensible sounds	2
	No response	1

PUPILS + Reactive − Nonreactive ± Sluggish

PUPIL GAUGE (MM)
2 3 4 5 6 7 8 9

EXTREMITIES

MOVEMENT	ABBREV.	STRENGTH	MOVEMENT	ABBREV.
VOLUNTARY	V	+STRONG	NONE	φ
COMMAND	C	−WEAK	DECORTICATE	Decor.
STIM/PURPOSEFUL	S	φABSENT	DECEREBRATE	Decer.
WITHDRAWS	W			

PULSES

A-ABSENT	W-WEAK	S-STRONG	D-DOPPLER

OBSTETRICAL LEGEND

BREAST:	S-SOFT	F-FIRM	E-ENGORGED
FUNDUS/PLACEMENT		S-SOFT	F-FIRM
LOCHIA:	S-SCANT	M-MODERATE	H-HEAVY
PERINEUM		C-CLEAN /	E-EDEMA

NS-49 (Rev. 5/95)

PAGE-1

(continues)

APPENDIX B–4 24-hour Progress Notes.
Reprinted with permission from Conroe Regional Medical Center Hospital, Conroe, Texas.

(continued)

PATIENT CARE RECORD

PATIENT-FAMILY TEACHING

TIME	PROBLEM #	PATIENT - FAMILY TEACHING	INITIAL

TIME	PROBLEM #	PSYCHOSOCIAL INTERVENTIONS / DC PLANNING	INITIAL

POST PARTUM ASSESSMENT (To be used on obstetrical patients only.)

DAY SHIFT		EVENING SHIFT		NIGHT SHIFT	
R **L**		**R** **L**		**R** **L**	
REFLEXES 1+ 2+ 3+ 4+ 1+ 2+ 3+ 4+		REFLEXES 1+ 2+ 3+ 4+ 1+ 2+ 3+ 4+		REFLEXES 1+ 2+ 3+ 4+ 1+ 2+ 3+ 4+	
CLONUS ABSENT ☐ ABSENT ☐		CLONUS ABSENT ☐ ABSENT ☐		CLONUS ABSENT ☐ ABSENT ☐	
PRESENT ___ BEATS PRESENT ___ BEATS		PRESENT ___ BEATS PRESENT ___ BEATS		PRESENT ___ BEATS PRESENT ___ BEATS	
HOMANS ABSENT ☐ ABSENT ☐		HOMANS ABSENT ☐ ABSENT ☐		HOMANS ABSENT ☐ ABSENT ☐	
PRESENT ☐ PRESENT ☐		PRESENT ☐ PRESENT ☐		PRESENT ☐ PRESENT ☐	

DAY SHIFT	EVENING SHIFT	NIGHT SHIFT
BREASTS SEE SOFT, TENDER, ENGORGED, FISSURES ☐ **NOTES**	**BREASTS** SEE SOFT, TENDER, ENGORGED, FISSURES ☐ **NOTES**	**BREASTS** SEE SOFT, TENDER, ENGORGED, FISSURES ☐ **NOTES**
FUNDUS FIRM, BOGGY LEVEL _____ BLADDER _____	**FUNDUS** FIRM, BOGGY LEVEL _____ BLADDER _____	**FUNDUS** FIRM, BOGGY LEVEL _____ BLADDER _____
PERINEUM - HEMORRHOIDS EPISIOTOMY - CLEAN, INTACT SWELLING, INFLAMMATION, DRAINAGE, HEMATOMA ☐ SEE NOTES	**PERINEUM - HEMORRHOIDS** EPISIOTOMY - CLEAN, INTACT SWELLING, INFLAMMATION, DRAINAGE, HEMATOMA ☐ SEE NOTES	**PERINEUM - HEMORRHOIDS** EPISIOTOMY - CLEAN, INTACT SWELLING, INFLAMMATION, DRAINAGE, HEMATOMA ☐ SEE NOTES
LOCHIA - VAG. DRAINAGE SM. - MED. - LARGE SEROSA - RUBRA - ALBA ☐ SEE NOTES	**LOCHIA - VAG. DRAINAGE** SM. - MED. - LARGE SEROSA - RUBRA - ALBA ☐ SEE NOTES	**LOCHIA - VAG. DRAINAGE** SM. - MED. - LARGE SEROSA - RUBRA - ALBA ☐ SEE NOTES
FEEDING SEE BREAST - BOTTLE - FOD ☐ NOTES	FEEDING SEE BREAST - BOTTLE - FOD ☐ NOTES	FEEDING SEE BREAST - BOTTLE - FOD ☐ NOTES
ROOMING IN YES - NO	**ROOMING IN** YES - NO	**ROOMING IN** YES - NO
BONDING POSITIVE - NEGATIVE	**BONDING** POSITIVE - NEGATIVE	**BONDING** POSITIVE - NEGATIVE
SIGNATURE TIME	SIGNATURE TIME	SIGNATURE TIME

PAGE-2

(continues)

(continued)

SEE CARE PLAN
NURSING DIAGNOSIS:

#		#		#	
	Airway Clearance, Ineffective		Grieving		Pain
	Anxiety		Home Maintenance Management, Impaired		Sensory/Perceptual Alt.
	Breathing Patterns, Ineffective		Hyperthermia		Skin Integrity, Impaired
	Cardiac Output, Decreased		Incontinence		Sleep Pattern Disturbance
	Communication, Impaired Verbal		Injury, High Risk for		Social Isolation
	Coping, Ineffective Individual		Knowledge Deficit		Thought Process, Altered
	Fatigue		Mobility, Impaired Physical		Tissue Perfusion, Alt.
	Fluid Vol., Alt. in		Nutrition, Alt. in		
	Gas Exchange, Impaired		Noncompliance		
					See Critical Pathway

TIME	PROB #	PT. OUTCOME / EVALUATION

INITIALS	SIGNATURES	INITIALS	SIGNATURES	INITIALS	SIGNATURES

(continues)

(continued)

NURSING INTERVENTION

		DAY / INITIAL	EVENING / INITIAL	NIGHT / INITIAL
D I E T		DIET: NPO REG. SOFT CLEAR LIQUID FULL LIQUIDS SPECIAL TYPE: _____ _____ FEED SELF, ASST. TOTAL _____ % DIET TAKEN SNACKS:	DIET: NPO REG. SOFT CLEAR LIQUID FULL LIQUIDS SPECIAL TYPE: _____ _____ FEED SELF, ASST. TOTAL _____ % DIET TAKEN SNACKS:	DIET: NPO REG. SOFT CLEAR LIQUID FULL LIQUIDS SPECIAL TYPE: _____ _____ FEED SELF, ASST. TOTAL _____ % DIET TAKEN SNACKS:
H Y G I E N E	☐ BED BATH ☐ TUB ☐ SHOWER ☐ SITZ	☐ NA ☐ SELF ☐ ASSIST ☐ COMPLETE	☐ NA ☐ SELF ☐ ASSIST ☐ COMPLETE	☐ NA ☐ SELF ☐ ASSIST ☐ COMPLETE
	HAIR/SHAVE	☐ YES ☐ NO	☐ YES ☐ NO	☐ YES ☐ NO
	ORAL CARE	☐ SELF ☐ COMPLETE ☐ ASSIST	☐ SELF ☐ COMPLETE ☐ ASSIST	☐ SELF ☐ COMPLETE ☐ ASSIST
	SKIN CARE	☐ NA ☐ SELF ☐ EGG CRATE ☐ ASSIST ☐ COMPLETE	☐ NA ☐ SELF ☐ EGG CRATE ☐ ASSIST ☐ COMPLETE	☐ NA ☐ SELF ☐ EGG CRATE ☐ ASSIST ☐ COMPLETE
	FOLEY CATH. CARE	☐ YES ☐ N/A	☐ YES ☐ N/A	☐ YES ☐ N/A
	DECUBITUS CARE	☐ YES ☐ N/A	☐ YES ☐ N/A	☐ YES ☐ N/A
	LINEN CHANGE	☐ YES ☐ NO	☐ YES ☐ NO	☐ YES ☐ NO
A C T I V I T Y	TYPE OF ACTIVITY	☐ BED ☐ CHAIR ☐ W/C ☐ AMB. ☐ DANGLE ☐ BRP ☐ ROM	☐ BED ☐ CHAIR ☐ W/C ☐ AMB. ☐ DANGLE ☐ BRP ☐ ROM	☐ BED ☐ CHAIR ☐ W/C ☐ AMB. ☐ DANGLE ☐ BRP ☐ ROM
	HOW ACCOMPLISHED	☐ SELF ☐ ASSIST ☐ PT ☐ WALKER ☐ CANE ☐ CRUTCH	☐ SELF ☐ ASSIST ☐ PT ☐ WALKER ☐ CANE ☐ CRUTCH	☐ SELF ☐ ASSIST ☐ PT ☐ WALKER ☐ CANE ☐ CRUTCH
	DEEP BREATHE AND COUGH	☐ Q2H ASSIST ☐ Q2H SELF @ ☐ IS@ ☐ N/A	☐ Q2H ASSIST ☐ Q2H SELF @ ☐ IS@ ☐ N/A	☐ Q2H ASSIST ☐ Q2H SELF @ ☐ IS@ ☐ N/A
	REST PERIOD POSITION/	☐ YES ☐ N/A ☐ Q2H ASSIST ☐ Q2H SELF @	☐ YES ☐ N/A ☐ Q2H ASSIST ☐ Q2H SELF @	
	REPOSITION	@ ☐ N/A	@ ☐ N/A	@ ☐ N/A
T R E A T M E N T S	NGT PLACEMENT CHECKED	☐ YES @ ☐ N/A	☐ YES @ ☐ N/A	☐ YES @ ☐ N/A
	FEEDING TUBE RESIDUAL (cc's)	☐ N/A cc's _____	☐ N/A cc's _____	☐ N/A cc's _____
	ORAL SUCTIONING	☐ YES @ ☐ N/A	☐ YES @ ☐ N/A	☐ YES @ ☐ N/A
	NASO-TRACH SUCTIONING	☐ YES @ ☐ N/A	☐ YES @ ☐ N/A	☐ YES @ ☐ N/A
	TRACH. CARE	☐ YES @ ☐ N/A	☐ YES @ ☐ N/A	☐ YES @ ☐ N/A
	FOLEY IRRIGATION	☐ YES @ ☐ N/A	☐ YES @ ☐ N/A	☐ YES @ ☐ N/A
	TRACTION	☐ YES TYPE _____ ☐ N/A	☐ YES TYPE _____ ☐ N/A	☐ YES TYPE _____ ☐ N/A
	ANTI-EMBOLIC STOCKINGS	☐ YES ☐ NO	☐ YES ☐ NO	☐ YES ☐ NO
	GUAIAC RESULT	☐ POS. ☐ Neg. _____	☐ POS. ☐ Neg. _____	☐ POS. ☐ Neg. lot# _____
	K-PAD	☐ YES LOCATION _____ ☐ N/A	☐ YES LOCATION _____ ☐ N/A	☐ YES LOCATION _____ ☐ N/A
	SUCTION	☐ YES LOCATION _____ ☐ N/A	☐ YES LOCATION _____ ☐ N/A	☐ YES LOCATION _____ ☐ N/A
I V	START/RESTART	BY	BY	BY
		TIME CATH SIZE	TIME CATH SIZE	TIME CATH SIZE
		# ATTEMPTS PUMP ☐ YES ☐ NO	# ATTEMPTS PUMP ☐ YES ☐ NO	# ATTEMPTS PUMP ☐ YES ☐ NO
		SITE	SITE	SITE
		# UNITS BLOOD	# UNITS BLOOD	# UNITS BLOOD
	TUBINGS CHANGED	☐ YES ☐ NO ☐ NA	☐ YES ☐ NO ☐ NA	☐ YES ☐ NO ☐ NA
S A F E T Y	BED CHECK	☐ YES ☐ NO ☐ N/A	☐ YES ☐ NO ☐ N/A	☐ YES ☐ NO ☐ N/A
	SIDE RAIL UP/ BED IN LOW POSITION	☐ X2 ☐ NO ☐ YES ☐ NO	☐ X2 ☐ NO ☐ YES ☐ NO	☐ X2 ☐ NO ☐ YES ☐ NO
	CALL BUTTON WITHIN REACH	☐ YES ☐ NO	☐ YES ☐ NO	☐ YES ☐ NO
	SEIZURE PRECAUTIONS	☐ N/A ☐ NO	☐ N/A ☐ NO	☐ N/A ☐ NO
	FALL HIGH RISK	☐ YES	☐ YES	☐ YES
	RESTRAINTS	☐ NO ☐ VEST ☐ WRIST ☐ ANKLE CHECK/REMOVED @ _____	☐ NO ☐ VEST ☐ WRIST ☐ ANKLE CHECK/REMOVED @ _____	☐ NO ☐ VEST ☐ WRIST ☐ ANKLE CHECK/REMOVED @ _____
	ISOLATION	☐ YES TYPE: _____ ☐ N/A	☐ YES TYPE: _____ ☐ N/A	☐ YES TYPE: _____ ☐ N/A
M I S C.	SPECIAL PREPS	☐ YES TYPE: _____ ☐ N/A	☐ YES TYPE: _____ ☐ N/A	☐ YES TYPE: _____ ☐ N/A
	SPECIMEN COLLECTED	☐ SENT TO LAB ☐ NA TYPE: _____	☐ SENT TO LAB ☐ NA TYPE: _____	☐ SENT TO LAB ☐ NA TYPE: _____
	SPECIMEN COLLECTED	☐ SENT TO LAB ☐ NA TYPE: _____	☐ SENT TO LAB ☐ NA TYPE: _____	☐ SENT TO LAB ☐ NA TYPE: _____
	PROCEDURE/DIAG. TEST			
	PHYSICIAN'S VISITS (NAME/TIME)			

(continues)

(continued)

PATIENT CARE RECORD

PATIENT ASSESSMENT

INSTRUCTIONS: CHECK □ OR FILL IN BLANKS AS APPROPRIATE

SHIFT ASSESSMENT	Time _____ DAY	Time _____ EVENING	Time _____ NIGHT
1. NEUROLOGICAL/ LEVEL OF CONSCIOUSNESS	□ ORIENTED □ DISORIENTED □ CONSCIOUS □ UNCONSCIOUS □ ALERT □ LETHARGIC □ SEDATED □ OTHER _____ PUPILS: □ EQUAL □ UNEQUAL □ DESCRIBE	□ ORIENTED □ DISORIENTED □ CONSCIOUS □ UNCONSCIOUS □ ALERT □ LETHARGIC □ SEDATED □ OTHER _____ PUPILS: □ EQUAL □ UNEQUAL □ DESCRIBE	□ ORIENTED □ DISORIENTED □ CONSCIOUS □ UNCONSCIOUS □ ALERT □ LETHARGIC □ SEDATED □ OTHER _____ PUPILS: □ EQUAL □ UNEQUAL □ DESCRIBE
2. PAIN	□ NO □ YES □ SEE NARRATIVE	□ NO □ YES □ SEE NARRATIVE	□ NO □ YES □ SEE NARRATIVE
3. EMOTIONAL BEHAVIOR	□ COOPERATIVE □ UNCOOPERATIVE □ COMBATIVE □ CALM □ ANXIOUS □ DEPRESSED □ UPSET □ ANGRY	□ COOPERATIVE □ UNCOOPERATIVE □ COMBATIVE □ CALM □ ANXIOUS □ DEPRESSED □ UPSET □ ANGRY	□ COOPERATIVE □ UNCOOPERATIVE □ COMBATIVE □ CALM □ ANXIOUS □ DEPRESSED □ UPSET □ ANGRY
4. RESPIRATORY	□ EVEN □ UNEVEN □ SOB □ LABORED □ SHALLOW □ DEEP BREATH SOUNDS CLEAR □ L □ R RALES □ L □ R RHONCI □ L □ R WHEEZES □ L □ R CONGESTED □ L □ R O₂ L/M □ NC □ MASK □ REBREATHER	□ EVEN □ UNEVEN □ SOB □ LABORED □ SHALLOW □ DEEP BREATH SOUNDS CLEAR □ L □ R RALES □ L □ R RHONCI □ L □ R WHEEZES □ L □ R CONGESTED □ L □ R O₂ L/M □ NC □ MASK □ REBREATHER	□ EVEN □ UNEVEN □ SOB □ LABORED □ SHALLOW □ DEEP BREATH SOUNDS CLEAR □ L □ R RALES □ L □ R RHONCI □ L □ R WHEEZES □ L □ R CONGESTED □ L □ R O₂ L/M □ NC □ MASK □ REBREATHER
5. GASTRO-INTESTINAL	BOWEL SOUNDS □ NORMAL □ ABSENT □ HYPERACTIVE □ HYPOACTIVE □ HOB↑_____° ABDOMINAL DISTENSION □ NO □ YES ABDO. CHARACTERISTICS □ SOFT □ FIRM □ RIGID NAUSEA: □ NO □ YES EMESIS □ NO □ YES EMESIS: #_____ , COLOR _____ STOOL: #_____ , CONSISTENCY _____ COLOR _____ NGT DRAINAGE □ NO □ YES COLOR _____ TUBE FEEDING TYPE _____ □ CONT RATE □ BOLUS CC'S @	BOWEL SOUNDS □ NORMAL □ ABSENT □ HYPERACTIVE □ HYPOACTIVE □ HOB↑_____° ABDOMINAL DISTENSION □ NO □ YES ABDO. CHARACTERISTICS □ SOFT □ FIRM □ RIGID NAUSEA: □ NO □ YES EMESIS □ NO □ YES EMESIS: #_____ , COLOR _____ STOOL: #_____ , CONSISTENCY _____ COLOR _____ NGT DRAINAGE □ NO □ YES COLOR _____ TUBE FEEDING TYPE _____ □ CONT RATE □ BOLUS CC'S @	BOWEL SOUNDS □ NORMAL □ ABSENT □ HYPERACTIVE □ HYPOACTIVE □ HOB↑_____° ABDOMINAL DISTENSION □ NO □ YES ABDO. CHARACTERISTICS □ SOFT □ FIRM □ RIGID NAUSEA: □ NO □ YES EMESIS □ NO □ YES EMESIS: #_____ , COLOR _____ STOOL: #_____ , CONSISTENCY _____ COLOR _____ NGT DRAINAGE □ NO □ YES COLOR _____ TUBE FEEDING TYPE _____ □ CONT RATE □ BOLUS CC'S @
6. INTEGUMENT	SKIN COLOR: □ NORMAL □ PALE □ CYANOTIC □ FLUSHED □ JAUNDICED □ MOTTLED SKIN CHARACTER: □ WARM □ COOL □ MOIST □ DRY SKIN TURGOR: _____ EDEMA □ NO □ YES SITE _____ IV/HEPARIN LOCK/SITE _____ CENTRAL LINE _____ DESCRIPTION: □ CLEAN □ ERYTHEMA □ EDEMA SOLUTION/RATE: _____	SKIN COLOR: □ NORMAL □ PALE □ CYANOTIC □ FLUSHED □ JAUNDICED □ MOTTLED SKIN CHARACTER: □ WARM □ COOL □ MOIST □ DRY SKIN TURGOR: _____ EDEMA □ NO □ YES SITE _____ IV/HEPARIN LOCK/SITE _____ CENTRAL LINE _____ DESCRIPTION: □ CLEAN □ ERYTHEMA □ EDEMA SOLUTION/RATE: _____	SKIN COLOR: □ NORMAL □ PALE □ CYANOTIC □ FLUSHED □ JAUNDICED □ MOTTLED SKIN CHARACTER: □ WARM □ COOL □ MOIST □ DRY SKIN TURGOR: _____ EDEMA □ NO □ YES SITE _____ IV/HEPARIN LOCK/SITE _____ CENTRAL LINE _____ DESCRIPTION: □ CLEAN □ ERYTHEMA □ EDEMA SOLUTION/RATE: _____
7. WOUND	LOCATION: _____ SIZE _____ APPEARANCE: _____ SKIN CLOSURE: _____ DRAINAGE: COLOR _____ AMT _____ DRESSING CHANGE # _____ DRAINS: TYPE SITE	LOCATION: _____ SIZE _____ APPEARANCE: _____ SKIN CLOSURE: _____ DRAINAGE: COLOR _____ AMT _____ DRESSING CHANGE # _____ DRAINS: TYPE SITE	LOCATION: _____ SIZE _____ APPEARANCE: _____ SKIN CLOSURE: _____ DRAINAGE: COLOR _____ AMT _____ DRESSING CHANGE # _____ DRAINS: TYPE SITE
8. GENITOURINARY	URINATING □ NO □ YES CLARITY _____ COLOR _____ INCONTINENT □ NO □ YES CATHETER: □ FOLEY □ STRAIGHT _____ c.c. GU IRRIGANT TYPE RATE	URINATING □ NO □ YES CLARITY _____ COLOR _____ INCONTINENT □ NO □ YES CATHETER: □ FOLEY □ STRAIGHT _____ c.c. GU IRRIGANT TYPE RATE	URINATING □ NO □ YES CLARITY _____ COLOR _____ INCONTINENT □ NO □ YES CATHETER: □ FOLEY □ STRAIGHT _____ c.c. GU IRRIGANT TYPE RATE
9. CARDIOVASCULAR	HEART: □ REGULAR □ IRREGULAR HEART SOUNDS: □ NORMAL □ ABNORMAL _____ TELEMETRY # RHYTHM	HEART: □ REGULAR □ IRREGULAR HEART SOUNDS: □ NORMAL □ ABNORMAL _____ TELEMETRY # RHYTHM	HEART: □ REGULAR □ IRREGULAR HEART SOUNDS: □ NORMAL □ ABNORMAL _____ TELEMETRY # RHYTHM
10. EXTREMITIES	□ FULL ROM ALL EXTREMITIES □ ROM DEFICITS: _____ □ RU □ LU □ RL □ LL PULSES: _____ RT. RADIAL □ NO □ YES LT. RADIAL □ NO □ YES RT. PEDALS □ NO □ YES LT. PEDALS □ NO □ YES	□ FULL ROM ALL EXTREMITIES □ ROM DEFICITS: _____ □ RU □ LU □ RL □ LL PULSES: _____ RT. RADIAL □ NO □ YES LT. RADIAL □ NO □ YES RT. PEDALS □ NO □ YES LT. PEDALS □ NO □ YES	□ FULL ROM ALL EXTREMITIES □ ROM DEFICITS: _____ □ RU □ LU □ RL □ LL PULSES: _____ RT. RADIAL □ NO □ YES LT. RADIAL □ NO □ YES RT. PEDALS □ NO □ YES LT. PEDALS □ NO □ YES
SIGNATURES AND INITIALS (ONE ONLY)	RN LVN	RN LVN	RN LVN

(continues)

(continued)

TIME/# NURSING PROGRESS NOTES / PATIENT OUTCOMES (CONT'D)

Conroe
Regional Medical Center

Interdisciplinary Patient/Family Education Record

PATIENT/FAMILY KNOWLEDGE DEFICIT

A
D
D
R
E
S
S
O
G
R
A
P
H

Init.	Signature & Title	Init.	Signature & Title

REFERENCE CODES:

Patient Educational Need/Problem	Discipline	Learning Barriers	Learner /Person Present	Teaching Method	Evaluation of Learning
1. Medication 2. Food & Drug Interaction 3. Equipment 4. Rehabilitation Techniques 5. Tests/Procedures 6. Surgery: Pre-op / Post-op 7. Nutrition Counseling 8. Responsibilities of patients in their care 9. Available commun. resources 10. Miscellaneous	N = Nursing RD = Dietitian CM = Case Manager Rx = Pharmacy SS = Social Worker RT = Resp. Therapist ST = Speech Therapy PT = Physical Therapy OT = Occup. Therapy HB = Hyperb. Wound O = Other	1. Language 2. Memory 3. Vision 4. Hearing 5. Fatigue/ Pain 6. Emotional 7. Ability to grasp concepts 8. Access to community resources 9. Financial Concerns 10 Religious Considerations 11. Motivation 12. Cultural Factors 13. Education Needs 14. Other age-related issues 15. None	P = Patient SP = Spouse M = Mother F = Father D = Daughter S = Son F = Friend SIG = Significant Other O = Other	1. Audiovisual 2. Demo. 3. Handout 4. Discussion 5. Class/lecture 6. Translator	1. Demo. w/o assistance 2. Demo with assistance 3. Needs additional teaching 4. Verbalizes understanding 5. Needs reinforcement 6. No evidence of understanding 7. Refer to other sources

OVERALL PATIENT/FAMILY EDUCATIONAL GOAL: Upon completion of teaching intervention, patient or family demonstrates &/or verbalizes understanding of identified needs or problems.

Patient Needs Problems	Team Intervention Use number of appropriate item(s)						Comments*	Problem Resolved	
Date	Need	Disci-pline	Barrier	Learner	Method	Eval-uation	Initial		Date	Initial

* Use asterisk to indicate further documentation in Progress Notes.

ptfmrec3

(continues)

APPENDIX B–5 Interdisciplinary Record.
Reprinted with permission from Conroe Regional Medical Center Hospital, Conroe, Texas.

(continued)

REFERENCE CODES:

Patient Educational Need/Problem	Discipline	Learning Barriers	Learner /Person Present	Teaching Method	Evaluation of Learning
1. Medication 2. Food & Drug Interaction 3. Equipment 4. Rehabilitation Techniques 5. Tests/Procedures 6. Surgery: Pre-op / Post-op 7. Nutrition Counseling 8. Responsibilities of patients in their care 9. Available commun. resources 10. Miscellaneous	N = Nursing RD = Dietitian CM = Case Manager Rx = Pharmacy SS = Social Worker RT = Resp. Therapist ST = Speech Therapy PT = Physical Therapy OT = Occup. Therapy HB = Hyperb. Wound O = Other	1. Language 2. Memory 3. Vision 4. Hearing 5. Fatigue/ Pain 6. Emotional 7. Ability to grasp concepts 8. Access to community resources 9. Financial Concerns 10 Religious Considerations 11. Motivation 12. Cultural Factors 13. Education Needs 14. Other age-related issues 15. None	P = Patient SP = Spouse M = Mother F = Father D = Daughter S = Son F = Friend SIG = Significant Other O = Other	1. Audiovisual 2. Demo. 3. Handout 4. Discussion 5. Class/lecture 6. Translator	1. Demo. w/o assistance 2. Demo with assistance 3. Needs additional teaching 4. Verbalizes understanding 5. Needs reinforcement 6. No evidence of understanding 7. Refer to other sources

Patient Needs Problems	Team Intervention Use number of appropriate item(s)						Comments*	Problem Resolved	
Date	Need	Discipline	Barrier	Learner	Method	Evaluation	Initial		Date	Initial

* Use asterisk to indicate further documentation in Progress Notes

GLOSSARY

KEY TERMS

Actual nursing diagnosis: a label approved by NANDA classifying specific client problems or needs

Analyze: the process of rationalizing, questioning, and classifying information to reach a conclusion about a client's needs

Assessment: the effect of gathering data, organizing the data, and then documenting the data

Auscultation: listening for sounds within the body, usually with a stethoscope

Baseline data: information initially collected, forming the client's database, used for future comparison

Care plan: written documentation of the second and third steps of the nursing process which cites the client's problems/needs, goals/outcomes of care, and nursing interventions to treat the problems/needs

Client centered: focused on the client

Closed question: communication technique consisting of questions that can be answered briefly with yes-or-no or one-word responses

Closure: the phase of the interview in which all information has been collected and summarized

Collaboration: an act of communicating with other disciplines/parties for the purpose of decision making or problem solving

Collaborative problem: monitoring for the onset of certain physiological risk complications

Confidentiality: nondisclosure of information obtained by the health care team about a client; this information is considered privileged and cannot be disclosed to a third party without the client's consent

Critical thinking: a purposeful, deliberate method of thinking used in search for meaning

Data clustering: technique used to group related or like data; helps determine relatedness of data; provides confirmation of existing problem

Decision making: a skill used throughout the nursing process; process of applying judgments based on systematic and scientific theories

Defining characteristics: clinical criteria representing the presence of diagnostic facts; signs and symptoms indicating a specific nursing diagnosis

Dependent nursing interventions: actions requiring an order from a physician or another health care professional

Diagnosis: classification of a disease, condition, or human response determined by scientific evaluation of signs and symptoms, history, and diagnostic studies

Discharge planning: planning that requires analysis of the client's present health status and anticipates the client's needs after discharge for continued care

Discontinue: to terminate the portion of the care plan once the client has achieved the goal

Documentation: the process of recording assessment data, the client's health status, care provided, and response to care; includes written evidence of the interactions between and among health care professionals, clients and their families, and health care organizations

Etiology: cause or condition most likely to be involved in the development of a problem

Evaluation: appraisal of results through judicious reasoning; the fifth step of the nursing process

Evaluative statement: written statement identifying the client's progress toward goal achievement and problem resolution

Expected outcome: probable results; a detailed statement describing methods through which a goal will be achieved

Focus charting: a documentation method which includes written evidence of data, action, and response (DAR)

Goal: broad aim, intent, or objective

Goal attainment: achieved when the subject of the goal demonstrates the stated behavior within the specified time frame

Holistic: caring for the total person, including physical, emotional, social, spiritual, and economic needs of the client

Implementation: the fourth step of the nursing process during which nursing interventions specified in the care plan are executed

Independent nursing interventions: nursing actions initiated by the nurse, not requiring direction or an order from another health care professional

Inspection: systematic process of observation, which includes visual examination of the external surface of the body, as well as its movements and posture

Interdependent nursing interventions: nursing actions developed in collaboration or consultation with other health care professionals to gain another's viewpoint

Interpret: analyze the meaning and its significance

Interview: a communication exchange between the client and nurse

Introduction phase: the phase of an interview in which the goals of the interview are stated

JCAHO: Joint Commission on Accreditation of Healthcare Organizations: a surveying body which certifies clinical and organization performance of an institution following established guidelines

Kardex: a condensed reference tool used during change-of-shift report and as a quick reference throughout the shift; this tool includes basic client care information

Long-term goal: goal that may not be achieved prior to discharge from care, but may require continued attention, usually over weeks to months

Measurable: able to be quantified

Medical diagnosis: illness, condition, or pathological state for which treatment is directed by a licensed physician

Modification: alteration or revision of original care plan

NANDA: North American Nursing Diagnosis Association, international group responsible for the development and refinement of nursing diagnoses

Narrative charting: a documentation method, for which the nurse records complete data relating to the client as progress notes, sometimes supplementing notes with flow sheets

Nursing diagnosis: a label approved by NANDA identifying specific client problems/needs; means of describing health problems which nurses are licensed to treat, including physical, sociological, or psychological; the process of identifying client problems and needs; recognized as the second step of the nursing process

Nursing interventions: prescriptions for specific actions to be carried out by nurses to promote, maintain, or restore health; specified activities executed by the nursing team that benefit the client in a predictable manner

Nursing process: an orderly, step-by-step, problem-solving method of providing nursing care; the five steps are assessment, diagnosis, planning, implementation, and evaluation

Objective data: what can be observed, measured, or felt by someone other than the person experiencing the phenomenon

Observation: skill of watching thoughtfully and deliberately using the senses, touch, sight, smell, and hearing

Open-ended question: interviewing technique that promotes client elaboration about a particular concern or problem

Palpation: process of examining by applying the hands or fingers to the external surface of the body to detect evidence of disease or abnormalities in organs

Percussion: physical examination technique that uses fingertips, cup of the hand, fist, or percussion hammer to hear sounds or feel vibrations

PIE charting: a method of documentation which includes written evidence of each problem, intervention, and evaluation

Planning: the third step of the nursing process, which includes identifying priority problems and interventions, setting realistic goals and expected outcomes, determining appropriate nursing interventions and scientific rationale, determining collaboration needs, and communicating the proposed care plan through documentation

Prioritize: to impose an order or rank of precedence

Priority: estimated to be more important

Problem: the identified label of a client's health problem or response to the medical condition or therapy for which nursing may intervene; also known as the nursing diagnosis

Problem solving: the procedure of deliberate, thoughtful steps instituted for data collection, problem identification, planning for resolution, execution of interventions

Problem statement: consists of the diagnostic label (NANDA nursing diagnosis), etiology or risk factor, and defining characteristics (if stating an actual problem)

Process: a series of planned actions or operations directed toward a particular result or goal

Rationale: the underlying reason behind a specific response

Reporting: includes verbal communication of facts regarding the client's health status and care being provided

Revision: the process of rewriting, amending, or improving

Risk nursing diagnosis: diagnostic label preceded by the phrase *risk for*; determined for potential problems the client is at risk for developing, where specific risk factors are present

Short-term goal: goal that usually must be met prior to discharge or progress to a less acute level of care; goal usually met within hours or days

Social communication: casual conversation, spontaneous and with no planned agenda

Strength: area of positive functioning in the client, used to support the care plan, such as the desire to maintain a healthy diet, family support, or desire to get well

Subjective data: symptom; what the client reports, believes, or feels

Therapeutic communication: conversation which is purposeful, goal-directed, focused on the client, and planned, creating a beneficial outcome for the client

Validation: the process of ascertaining that data are factual

Verification: process of providing confirmation or proof

Wellness diagnosis: a judgment based upon a client's transition from a specific level of health to a higher level of health

Wellness nursing diagnosis: diagnostic label preceded by the phrase *potential for enhanced*, determined when a client has indicated a desire to attain a higher level of wellness in a particular area

Working phase: the phase of the interview that focuses on data collection

BIBLIOGRAPHY

Ackley, Betty J., & Ladwig, Gail B. (1997). *Nursing diagnosis handbook: A guide to planning care* (3rd ed.). St. Louis, MO: Mosby-Year Book.

Alfaro-LeFevre, Rosalinda. (1998). *Applying nursing process: A step-by-step guide* (4th ed.). Philadelphia: J.B. Lippincott.

American Nurses Association. (1991). *Standards of clinical nursing practice*. Washington, DC: Author.

Benner, P. (1984). *From novice to expert*. Menlo Park, CA: Addison-Wesley Publishers.

Carpenito, Lynda Juall. (1997a). *Handbook of nursing diagnosis* (7th ed.). Philadelphia: J.B. Lippincott.

Carpenito, Lynda Juall. (1997b). *Nursing diagnosis: Application to clinical practice* (7th ed.). Philadelphia: Lippincott-Raven.

DeLaune, Sue C., & Ladner, Patricia K. (1998). *Fundamentals of nursing: Standards and practice*. New York: Delmar Publishers.

Doenges, Marilynn E., & Moorhouse, Mary Frances. (1998). *Nurse's pocket guide: Diagnoses, interventions, and rationales* (6th ed.). Philadelphia: F.A. Davis Company.

Nightingale, Florence. (1946). *Notes on nursing: What it is, and what it is not*. Philadelphia: Edward Stern & Company.

North American Nursing Diagnosis Association. (1999). *Nursing diagnosis: Definitions and classifications 1999–2000*. Philadelphia: Author.

Shaw, Michael (Ed.). (1998). *Charting made incredibly easy*. Springhouse, PA: Springhouse.

Thomas, Clayton L. (Ed.). (1993). *Taber's cyclopedic medical dictionary* (17th ed.). Philadelphia: F. A. Davis Company.

Wilkinson, Judith M. (2000). *Nursing diagnosis handbook with NIC interventions and NOC outcomes* (7th ed.). Upper Saddle River, NJ: Prentice-Hall, Inc.